Essentials of ENT

A Practical Guide for Medical Students and Junior Doctors

Dr. Shaun M. Olson, MD, FACS

Copyright © 2024 by Dr. Shaun M. Olson.
All rights reserved. No part of this book may be reproduced, stored in a retrieval system, or transmitted in any form or by any means, electronic, mechanical, photocopying, recording, or otherwise, without prior written permission from the publisher, except for brief quotations used in reviews or scholarly works.

Acknowledgements

I would like to express my deepest gratitude to all those who contributed to the creation of Essentials of ENT: A Practical Guide for Medical Students and Junior Doctors. First and foremost, I extend my thanks to my colleagues, mentors, and educators who have shared their invaluable knowledge and experience in the field of ENT. Their guidance has been instrumental in shaping my understanding and passion for this specialty.

I am also grateful to my family for their unwavering support and encouragement throughout the writing process. Their patience and belief in me have been a constant source of motivation.

Special thanks to the medical students, junior doctors, and healthcare professionals whose insights and feedback have enriched this book, ensuring it remains practical and relevant to those embarking on their medical journeys.

Finally, my sincere appreciation goes to the publishers and editorial team for their dedication and professionalism in bringing this work to fruition.

This book is the result of collaborative effort, and I am deeply thankful to all who have contributed to its success.

Preface

The field of Ear, Nose, and Throat (ENT) medicine is as vast and intricate as it is essential to the overall health and well-being of our patients. As medical students and junior doctors embark on their clinical journeys, they are often confronted with the complexities of diagnosing and managing conditions that span a wide range of pathologies. From the simple sore throat to life-threatening head and neck cancers, the role of the ENT specialist is indispensable.

Essentials of ENT: A Practical Guide for Medical Students and Junior Doctors has been carefully crafted to address the needs of those entering this field or expanding their clinical expertise in otolaryngology. This book serves as both a comprehensive introduction and a practical reference, designed to guide you through the core concepts and essential clinical practices of ENT care. Whether you are beginning your studies in this specialty or are already involved in clinical rotations, this guide provides the fundamental knowledge and skills you will need to navigate the complexities of ENT medicine with confidence and clarity.

As you progress through this book, you will find that it balances theory and practice, equipping you with not only an understanding of the anatomical and physiological foundations of ENT medicine but also with the tools to diagnose, treat, and manage a broad spectrum of disorders affecting the ear, nose, and throat. This text covers a variety of common and complex conditions, ranging from hearing impairment, sinus diseases, and nasal obstructions, to voice disorders, throat cancers, and pediatric ENT concerns.

The focus of Essentials of ENT is on practical knowledge that can be immediately applied in clinical settings. Each chapter is designed to build your understanding step by step, offering clear explanations of the mechanisms behind ENT conditions, diagnostic procedures, and treatment protocols. Throughout the book, you will find clinical tips, illustrations, and real-world case scenarios to aid in honing your clinical reasoning and decision-making skills.

An integral aspect of this book is the emphasis on both the medical and surgical aspects of ENT care. The treatment options for many ENT conditions span a spectrum from conservative management to surgical interventions. For the aspiring physician or surgeon, this book outlines the indications, techniques, and post-operative care for common ENT surgeries. It is my belief that a thorough understanding of both the medical and surgical approaches is essential for delivering the best care to our patients.

Furthermore, the dynamic and multidisciplinary nature of ENT care requires effective communication, particularly when coordinating with other specialties. As you will see throughout this guide, an understanding of the role of the ENT specialist in a collaborative healthcare team is paramount to achieving optimal patient outcomes.

This book is not only intended as a reference for students and junior doctors but also as a resource for healthcare providers who wish to refresh or solidify their knowledge of ENT practices. As you grow in your clinical practice, the foundational knowledge contained in these pages will serve as a touchstone for continued learning and professional development.

As you embark on your journey through the world of ENT, remember that the nuances of this specialty are best learned through patient care. The skills and knowledge you will gain here are meant to complement your hands-on experience, which is the cornerstone of your medical education. I hope that this guide serves as a valuable resource to support your learning and growth in ENT, and that it instills in you a deep appreciation for the critical role the ear, nose, and throat play in human health.

It has been an honor to contribute this work, and I trust that it will provide you with the knowledge and confidence to become a skilled and compassionate healthcare provider, ready to care for patients with a wide variety of ENT conditions.

With best wishes for your success and continued learning,

Dr. Shaun M. Olson, MD, FACS

Acknowledgments
Preface
Table of Contents
List of Abbreviations

Table of contents

Introduction to ENT
Overview of ENT Anatomy and Physiology
Common ENT Conditions and Their Clinical Importance
Approach to History Taking and Examination in ENT

Neck Dissection
Indications for Neck Dissection
Types of Neck Dissection: Selective, Modified Radical, Radical, and Extended Radical
Surgical Techniques and Protocols
Consent and Postoperative Complications

Surgical Tracheostomy
Definition and Clinical Applications

Indications for Elective and Emergency Tracheostomy
Step-by-Step Surgical Technique
Perioperative and Postoperative Care
Complications and Their Management

Airway Emergencies in ENT
Recognition and Initial Management
Role of Tracheostomy in Airway Obstruction
Case Studies on ENT Emergencies

Advanced ENT Procedures
Endoscopic Sinus Surgery
Tonsillectomy and Adenoidectomy
Cochlear Implantation: Indications and Outcomes

Common ENT Infections and Their Management
Otitis Media and Externa
Sinusitis: Acute and Chronic
Pharyngitis and Laryngitis

Head and Neck Oncology

Overview of Common Malignancies
Diagnostic Approaches
Multidisciplinary Treatment Strategies

Pediatric ENT
Common Pediatric ENT Conditions
Special Considerations in Surgical and Medical Management

Audiology and Hearing Disorders
Basics of Audiological Testing
Management of Hearing Loss
Assistive Devices and Surgical Interventions

ENT Trauma
Management of Nasal, Ear, and Throat Injuries
Principles of Emergency Care and Reconstruction

ENT Equipment and Instrumentation
Overview of Tools Used in ENT Practice
Operative and Outpatient Applications

Case-Based Learning

Clinical Scenarios for Practical Application Problem-Solving and Decision-Making in ENT

List of Abbreviations

1. **AOM** – Acute Otitis Media

2. **CT** – Computed Tomography

3. **EEG** – Electroencephalogram

4. **ENT** – Ear, Nose, and Throat

5. **FESS** – Functional Endoscopic Sinus Surgery

6. **FNA** – Fine Needle Aspiration

7. **GCS** – Glasgow Coma Scale

8. **HNSCC** – Head and Neck Squamous Cell Carcinoma

9. **MRI** – Magnetic Resonance Imaging

10. **NICE** – National Institute for Health and Care Excellence

11. **OAE** – Otoacoustic Emissions

12. **OSA** – Obstructive Sleep Apnea

13. **PVD** – Peripheral Vascular Disease

14. **PTA** – Pure Tone Audiometry

15. **RT** – Radiotherapy

16. **SCC** – Squamous Cell Carcinoma

17. **TTS** – Tympanoplasty Tube Surgery

18. **TM** – Tympanic Membrane

19. **TMD** – Temporomandibular Disorder

20. **VNG** – Videonystagmography

Glossary of ENT Terminology

General ENT History: A Structured Approach for Clinical Practice

Introduction to History Taking in ENT

Effective history-taking is a fundamental skill that underpins all stages of medical training and practice. Establishing a good rapport with the patient not only fosters trust but also facilitates a thorough exploration of their symptoms, concerns, and expectations. By the conclusion of a detailed history, you should have a clear sense of potential differential diagnoses, laying the foundation for targeted clinical evaluation.

Preparation Before Beginning

Hygiene: Wash your hands thoroughly.

Introduction: Introduce yourself to the patient and ensure they are at ease.

Engagement: Maintain good eye contact and build rapport, including with parents or caregivers if present.

Structured Framework for ENT History Taking

1. Presenting Complaint (PC):

Begin with an open question: "What brings you here today?"

2. History of Presenting Complaint (HPC):

Probe the onset, duration, and progression: "When did this issue start?"

Explore specific risk factors and relevant details, tailored to the presenting issue (e.g., ear, nose, or throat).

Refer to condition-specific guidance for targeted questions.

3. Previous Episodes:

Investigate frequency, severity, response to past treatments, and history of hospitalizations.

4. Past Medical History (PMH):

Review relevant medical conditions, especially those affecting ENT health.

5. Birth History:

Particularly relevant for pediatric patients with ear-related issues.

6. Drug History (DH):

Document current medications, including over-the-counter drugs and vaccinations.

7. Allergies:

Inquire about drug or environmental allergies and any associated reactions.

8. Family History:

Assess for hereditary conditions or familial predispositions.

9. Social History (SH):

Evaluate the impact of the complaint on daily life and quality of living.

10. Systemic Review:

Check for bleeding tendencies, bruising, or systemic conditions that may affect ENT health.

Concluding the History

Summary: Recap the patient's history to confirm your understanding.

Clarifications: Ask if there is any additional information they wish to share.

Comprehensive Guide to Ear Examination

Preparation Before the Examination

Hand Hygiene: Wash or sanitize your hands thoroughly.

Introduce Yourself: Greet the patient and explain the procedure to ensure they are comfortable and informed.

Assess Pain: Ask about any pain, tenderness, or discomfort in the ears.

Patient Positioning:

Adults: Position the patient in a chair and stand at their side for easy access.

Children: Position them on a caregiver's lap. The caregiver should gently secure the child's head and arms for stability while incorporating play to reduce anxiety.

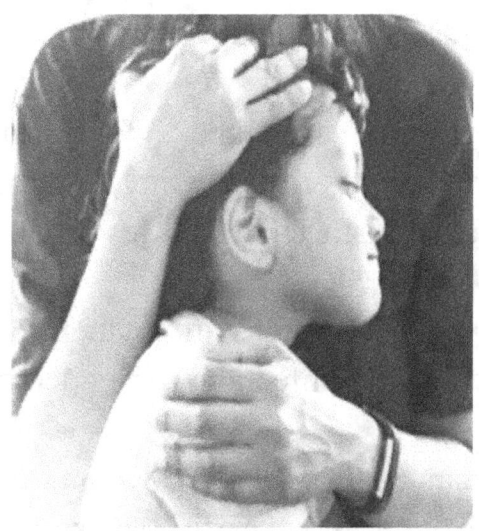

Fig. 1: Proper Child Positioning for Ear Examination

Inspection

1. General Inspection:

Observe from the front: Evaluate the size, symmetry, and appearance of the pinnae. Look for abnormalities such as protrusion or congenital deformities (e.g., microtia).

2. Detailed Ear Examination:

Preauricular Area: Check for scars (e.g., post-parotidectomy), swelling, redness, or congenital anomalies like sinuses or pits.

Pinna: Assess for signs of erythema, swelling (e.g., haematoma, infection), or tenderness.

Post-auricular Area: Move the pinna forward to inspect behind the ear for scars or swelling suggestive of infections like mastoiditis.

3. Sequential Examination: Always start with the unaffected ear to establish a baseline for comparison.

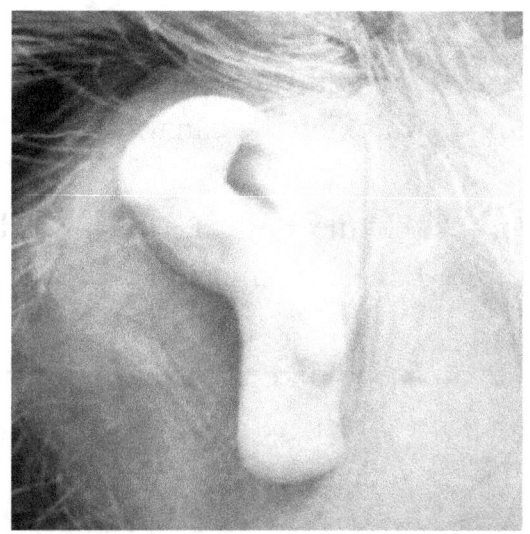

Fig. 2: Congenital Microtia of the External Ear Canal

Otoscopy

1. Equipment: Use an otoscope with adequate magnification and illumination. Select the largest speculum that comfortably fits the external auditory canal (EAC).

2. Technique:

Adults: Gently pull the pinna upwards and backward to straighten the canal.

Children: Pull the pinna downwards and backward for better visualization.

Hold the otoscope like a pencil, resting your little finger on the cheek to prevent injury if the patient moves suddenly.

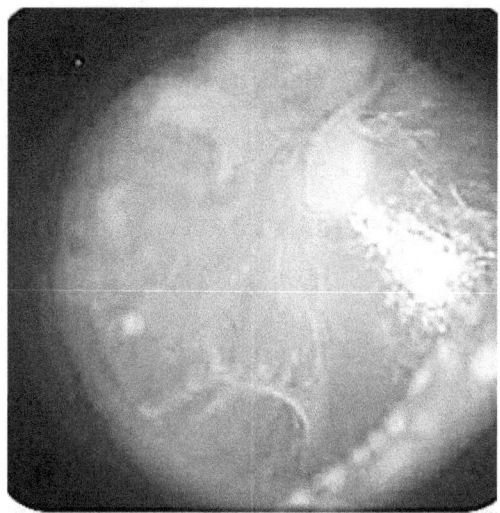

Fig. 3: Healthy Right Tympanic Membrane

3. Findings:

External Auditory Canal: Look for wax, discharge, redness, or swelling.

Tympanic Membrane: Check for the light reflex in the anteroinferior quadrant. Assess color (normal is grey and translucent), position (retracted, bulging), and integrity (perforation, tympanosclerosis).

Ossicles: Identify visible structures such as the malleus and incus.

Pneumatic Otoscopy: Test tympanic membrane mobility to assess for fluid or infection in the middle ear.

Hearing Assessment

1. General Observation: Note whether the patient can hear conversational speech or is using a hearing aid.

2. Free Field Speech Testing:

Perform at varying distances and intensities (whisper, conversational tone, loud voice).

Use masking techniques to ensure accurate assessment.

Correlate findings with approximate hearing thresholds (e.g., whisper at 60 cm suggests hearing better than 30 dB).

3. Tuning Fork Tests:

Weber's Test: Place a vibrating tuning fork on the midline of the forehead or head apex. Ask the patient to identify where the sound is louder.

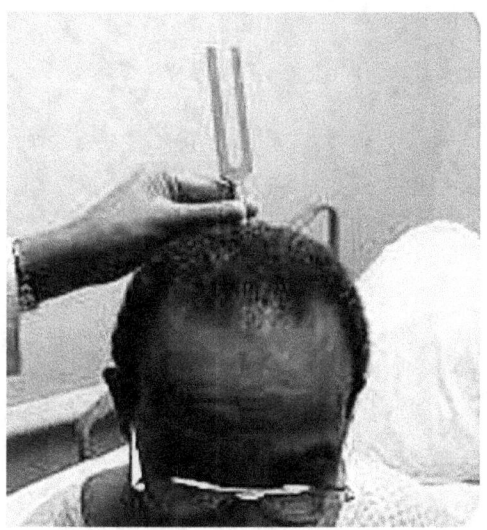

Fig. 4: Weber Test

Interpretation:

Louder in one ear indicates conductive hearing loss in that ear or sensorineural loss in the opposite ear.

Rinne's Test: Compare bone conduction (tuning fork on mastoid) to air conduction (tuning fork near the ear canal).

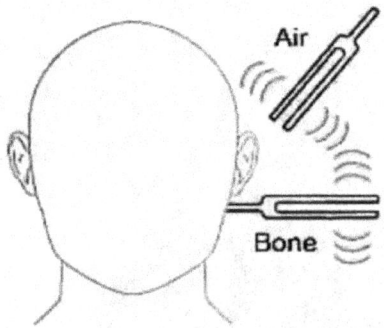

Fig. 5: Rinne's test

Interpretation:

Positive Rinne (AC > BC): Normal or sensorineural hearing loss.

Negative Rinne (BC > AC): Conductive hearing loss.

Facial Nerve Examination

Include a detailed assessment of facial nerve function, referencing the cranial nerve examination section for technique.

Concluding the Examination

1. Thank the patient and address any concerns.

2. Perform hand hygiene.

3. If in a clinical exam setting, summarize findings and propose additional investigations, such as:

Nasendoscopy: To evaluate nasopharyngeal conditions like adenoids or carcinoma.

Pure Tone Audiometry: For detailed hearing assessment.

Tympanometry: To evaluate middle ear function.

Comprehensive Guide to ENT and Thyroid Examination

Facial Nerve Examination

Refer to the "Cranial Nerves Examination" section for detailed guidance.

Concluding the Exam:

Thank the patient.

Wash your hands thoroughly.

If in an exam setting, summarize your findings to the examiner and discuss further investigations, such as:

Rigid Nasendoscopy: Helps identify nasopharyngeal conditions like adenoids or carcinoma.

Pure Tone Audiometry and Tympanometry: Useful for evaluating hearing and middle ear function.

Nasal Examination

Preparation

1. Wash and sanitize your hands.

2. Introduce yourself and explain the procedure to the patient.

3. Obtain consent and ensure the patient is comfortable in a well-lit environment.

4. Ask about:

Pain or tenderness.

Previous surgeries.

Inspection

1. Frontal View: Assess for:

Shape and deviations from the midline.

Symmetry between sides.

Scars or skin changes.

Divide the nose into thirds for better description:

Upper third (bony vault).

Middle third (dorsal septum and upper lateral cartilages).

Lower third (nasal tip and soft tissues).

2. Lateral View: Examine:

Shape (e.g., humps, collapse).

Projection and tip rotation (upward or downward).

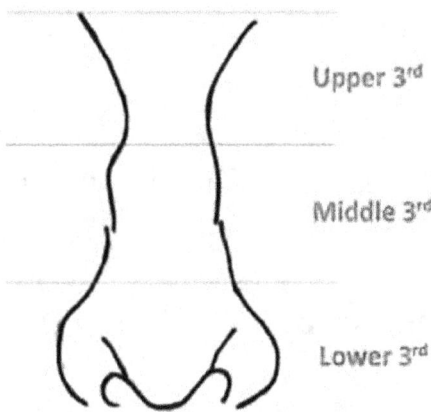

Fig. 6: Upper, middle and lower thirds of the nose

3. Inferior View: Check for:

Symmetry.

Deviations.

Scars from prior surgery.

Palpation

Skin: Assess thickness (thin over bone, thicker over the lower nose).

Tip Recoil: Gently press the nasal tip to evaluate resistance, indicating tip support integrity.

Anterior Rhinoscopy

Use a Thudicum's speculum and headlight for examination. Ensure alignment of the light source with the nasal cavity.

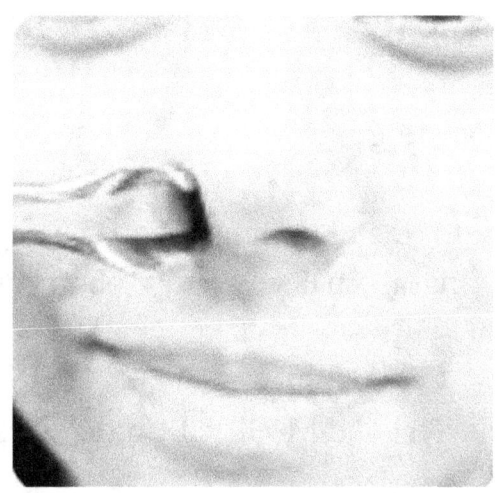

Fig. 7: How to perform anterior rhinoscopy with a Thudicum's speculum.

Common findings include:

Septal deviations.

Swelling (e.g., rhinitis with enlarged turbinates).

Septal perforations or prominent blood vessels.

Nasal polyps.

Additional Tests

1. Nasal Misting:

Use a cold metal tongue depressor to assess bilateral nasal patency by observing mist formation.

2. Cottle's Test and Modified Cottle's Test:

Assess external/internal nasal valve patency and detect nasal airway narrowing.

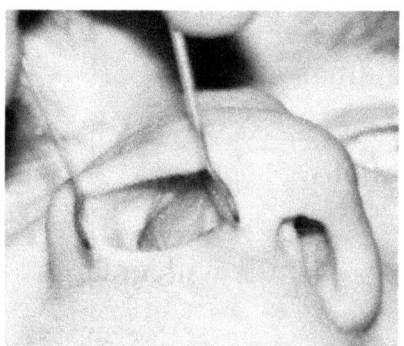

Fig. 8: Rightward Septal Deviation

Neck and Thyroid Examination

Preparation

1. Wash hands.

2. Introduce yourself and explain the procedure.

3. Ensure patient comfort and proper exposure of the neck (ideally up to the clavicles).

4. Confirm mobility for thorough assessment.

Inspection

Assess the neck from the front and sides for:

Asymmetry or masses.

Scars from prior surgeries.

Skin changes, such as radiotherapy effects or swelling.

Palpation

Use fingertips for sensitivity.

Examine from behind the patient, rolling tissues gently.

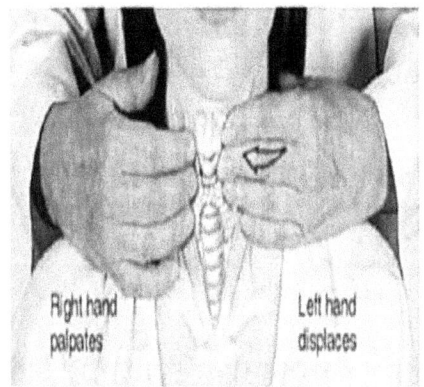

Fig. 9: Proper Hand Placement for Thyroid Exam

Ask the patient to:

Swallow water (thyroid origin lumps move upward).

Stick out their tongue (midline lumps moving up suggest thyroglossal cysts).

Lymph Node Assessment

Start with submental lymph nodes, progressing to submandibular, pre/post-auricular, occipital, anterior/posterior cervical chain, and supraclavicular nodes.

Thyroid Palpation

Detects characteristics like tenderness, temperature, texture, mobility, size, and consistency of nodules.

Additional Tests

1. Percussion: Tap over the sternum for retrosternal goitres.

2. Auscultation: Listen for bruits indicating increased blood flow, often associated with hyperthyroidism.

3. Pemberton's Test: Positive if raising the arms causes venous congestion or a hoarse voice.

General Thyroid Status Examination

1. Hands:

Check for tremors (hyperthyroidism).

Assess for thyroid acropachy, palmar erythema, or sweating.

Measure pulse (tachycardia, bradycardia, or atrial fibrillation).

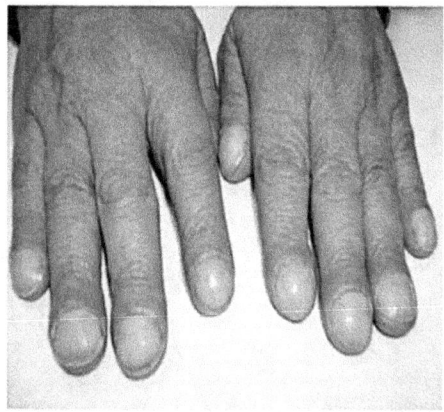

Fig. 10: Thyroid-Related Acropachy

2. Face:

Look for "peaches and cream" complexion (hypothyroidism).

Examine eyebrows for thinning (loss of outer third in hypothyroidism).

Assess for Graves' ophthalmopathy (proptosis, lid lag).

3. Legs:

Inspect for pretibial myxedema.

Check reflexes (brisk in hyperthyroidism, slow in hypothyroidism).

Concluding the Examination

1. Thank the patient.

2. Wash hands thoroughly.

3. Summarize findings to the examiner.

4. Suggest further investigations if needed, such as flexible nasendoscopy or imaging studies.

Comprehensive Guide to Cranial Nerve Examination

Preparation

1. Introduction and Consent: Introduce yourself to the patient and explain the procedure. Obtain informed consent.

2. Hygiene: Perform hand hygiene to maintain aseptic conditions.

3. Assessment of Pain or Tenderness: Ask if the patient is experiencing any tenderness or discomfort before starting the examination.

Cranial Nerve I: Olfactory Nerve

Informal Testing: Ask the patient if they have noticed any changes in their sense of smell.

Formal Testing: Use a validated smelling test, such as the University of Pennsylvania Smell Identification Test (UPSIT), for precise assessment.

Cranial Nerves II, III, IV, VI: Optic, Oculomotor, Trochlear, and Abducens Nerves

Vision and Eye Movements:

Inspect for normal color vision and smooth eye movements.

Abnormalities may indicate conditions like skull base tumors or orbital infections.

Clinical Example: Gradenigo's syndrome presents with unilateral periorbital pain, diplopia (from CN VI palsy), and petrositis, often secondary to acute otitis media.

Cranial Nerve V: Trigeminal Nerve

1. Motor Component:

Ask the patient to clench their teeth while palpating the masseter and temporalis muscles to assess tone.

Observe mouth opening for any deviation, which tests the function of the pterygoid muscles.

2. Sensory Component:

With the patient's eyes closed, lightly touch their forehead, cheeks, and jaw bilaterally using cotton wool. Ask them to confirm when they feel the touch.

Assess the ophthalmic, maxillary, and mandibular divisions. Temperature and pain sensation are rarely tested unless indicated.

3. Reflex Testing:

Corneal Reflex: The afferent limb involves CN V, while the efferent limb involves CN VII.

Jaw Jerk Reflex: Minimal or absent is normal. A brisk response suggests pathology, except in some younger patients where it may be normal.

Cranial Nerve VII: Facial Nerve

1. Inspection: Evaluate facial tone and symmetry.

2. Motor Assessment: Test facial movements to assess the branches of the facial nerve:

Raise eyebrows (forehead wrinkling).

Close your eyes tightly.

Puff cheeks, smile, and show teeth.

3. Special Features:

Hyperacusis indicates a lesion affecting the nerve to stapedius.

Taste loss suggests tympani involvement.

Cranial Nerve VIII: Vestibulocochlear Nerve

1. Hearing Assessment:

Use free-field testing or whisper tests.

Perform Weber and Rinne tests to differentiate conductive and sensorineural hearing loss.

Confirm findings with pure-tone audiometry if necessary.

Cranial Nerves IX and X: Glossopharyngeal and Vagus Nerves

1. Oral Examination:

Ask the patient to open their mouth and say "ahh." Note any uvular deviation (deviates away from the lesion).

2. Voice and Cough:

Assess for hoarseness or bovine cough, which could indicate recurrent laryngeal nerve palsy.

3. Swallowing and Gag Reflex: Evaluate swallowing ability and test the gag reflex if clinically indicated.

Cranial Nerve XI: Accessory Nerve

Ask the patient to shrug their shoulders against resistance to test the trapezius muscles.

Assess the ability to turn the head against resistance, which evaluates the contralateral sternocleidomastoid muscle.

Cranial Nerve XII: Hypoglossal Nerve

1. Tongue Examination:

Inspect for atrophy or fasciculations.

Ask the patient to protrude their tongue; deviation occurs towards the side of the lesion.

2. Motor Function: Instruct the patient to move their tongue side to side.

Conclusion

1. Thank the patient for their cooperation.

2. Perform hand hygiene after the examination.

3. Summarize your findings clearly and communicate them to the relevant team members or documentation.

Anatomy of the Ear

The ear is anatomically divided into three primary sections:

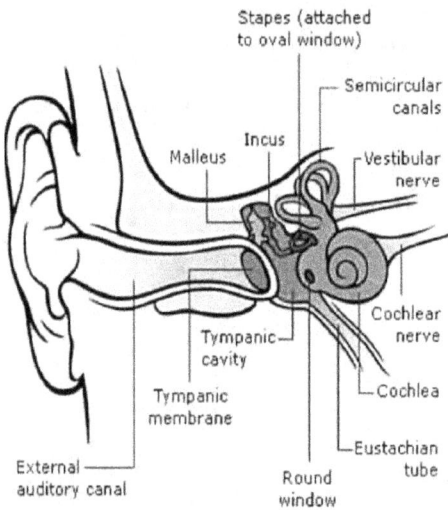

Fig. 11: External Auditory Canal and Middle Ear Structure

1. External Ear

2. Middle Ear

3. Inner Ear

External Ear

The external ear comprises the pinna (auricle) and the external auditory canal.

Pinna (Auricle):

The pinna is made up of elastic cartilage, shaped into various folds, and features a fibrofatty lobule (see Fig. 12).

Its nerve supply includes the greater auricular nerve, lesser occipital nerve, and branches of the facial nerve.

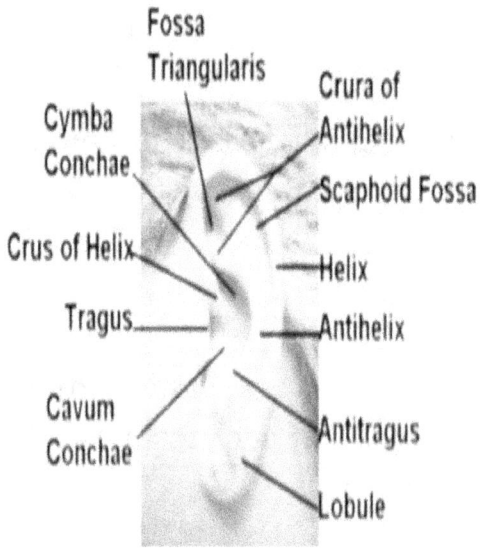

Fig. 12: External Ear and Middle Ear Anatomy

Nerve Supply and Anatomy of the Pinna and External Auditory Canal

Nerve Supply of the Pinna

Lateral Surface:

Anterosuperior Region: Supplied by the auriculotemporal nerve (branch of V3).

Anteroinferior Region: Innervated by the great auricular nerve (C2/3).

Posterior Region: Supplied by the lesser occipital nerve (C2).

Conchal Bowl and Ear Canal: Innervated by the auricular branch of the vagus nerve.

Medial Surface:

Primarily innervated by the greater auricular nerve (C2/3) and the lesser occipital nerve (C2).

External Auditory Canal (EAC)

The external auditory canal is an oblique tube approximately 3 cm in length:

Outer One-Third: Composed of cartilage and contains ceruminous glands responsible for wax production.

Inner Two-Thirds: Composed of bone, leading medially to the tympanic membrane, which forms the canal's medial boundary.

Clinical Note – Examining the EAC:

Adults: The canal is angled superiorly and posteriorly in the outer third and inferiorly and anteriorly in the inner two-thirds. To examine the canal, pull the auricle superiorly and posteriorly to align these sections.

Infants: Gently pull the pinna posteriorly.

Blood Supply of the External Ear

Auriculotemporal Branch: From the superficial temporal artery.

Posterior Auricular Branch: From the external carotid artery.

Clinical Relevance – Cauliflower Ear

The cartilage of the ear relies on the overlying perichondrium for nutrition. Trauma can cause separation between these layers, often filled with blood, infection, or inflammation. This can result in cartilage necrosis and subsequent deformity known as a cauliflower ear (refer to Fig. 13).

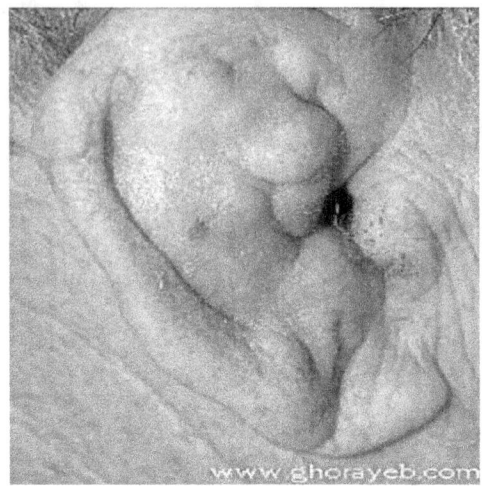

Fig. 13: Cauliflower Ear

Nerve Supply of the External Ear Canal

The external ear canal receives its nerve supply from:

Auriculotemporal nerve (branch of V3)

Auricular branch of the vagus nerve

The Middle Ear

The middle ear is an air-filled cavity within the temporal bone, lined with a mucous membrane. It communicates with the nasopharynx via the Eustachian tube and primarily functions to amplify and transmit sound energy.

Boundaries and Features:

Lateral Boundary: The tympanic membrane, a circular structure approximately 1 cm in diameter, forms the lateral boundary.

Innervation: Outer surface by the auriculotemporal nerve and auricular branch of the vagus nerve.

Appearance: Normally greyish-pink when healthy.

Cone Reflex: When viewed through an otoscope, its concavity produces a cone of light in the anteroinferior quadrant.

Umbo: The deepest point of concavity where the handle of the malleus attaches, serving as the origin of the cone of light.

Pars Flaccida: The thin, flexible part critical to cholesteatoma pathophysiology.

Pars Tensa: The more rigid, remaining portion of the tympanic membrane.

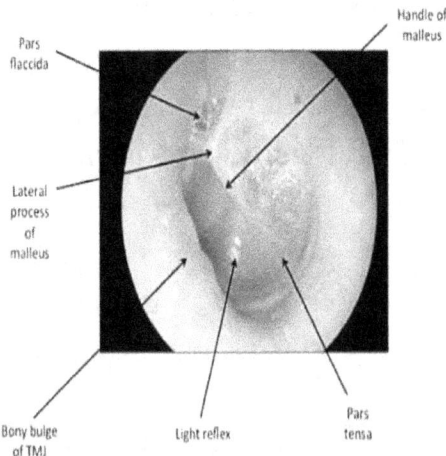

Fig. 14: Labeled Diagram of the Left Tympanic Membrane

Ossicles:

The middle ear contains three ossicles:

1. Malleus (largest):

The lateral process attaches to the tympanic membrane.

The head articulates with the body of the incus.

2. Incus:

The long process connects to the head of the stapes.

3. Stapes:

Consists of two limbs (anterior and posterior crus) attached to the oval window's footplate.

Associated Structures:

Muscles:

Tensor tympani and stapedius regulate ossicle movement.

Chorda Tympani: Provides taste sensation to the anterior two-thirds of the tongue.

Facial Nerve: Passes through the middle ear, with clinical significance in conditions like facial nerve palsy.

The Inner Ear: Structure, Function, and Clinical Relevance

Anatomy and Location

The inner ear is situated within the petrous part of the temporal bone, positioned medial to the middle ear.

Functions

Cochlea: Converts sound waves into electrical signals that the brain processes and interprets.

Semicircular Canals (superior, lateral, posterior): Detect angular head movements.

Utricle and Saccule: Sense linear accelerations—forward/backward for the utricle and up/down for the saccule.

Clinical Insights

Auditory Sensitivity: Humans typically detect sounds between 20 and 20,000 Hz.

Cochlear Tonotopy: High-frequency sounds are sensed at the cochlear base, while low-frequency sounds are detected at the apex. Age-related hearing loss (presbycusis) often reduces high-frequency detection.

Dizziness and Vertigo: Evaluation and Management

Overview

True Vertigo: Perceived spinning of the environment, distinct from general dizziness or disequilibrium.

Epidemiology

Predominantly affects females, with a male-to-female ratio of 1:3.

Causes and Differentiation

Understanding vertigo's duration and frequency is key to distinguishing peripheral (ear-related) from central (brain-related) causes.

Peripheral Causes:

Benign Paroxysmal Positional Vertigo (BPPV): Most common cause; onset typically between ages 40–60.

Vestibular Neuronitis: Continuous vertigo lasting over 24 hours, often with nausea.

Meniere's Disease: Characterized by episodic vertigo, fluctuating low-frequency hearing loss, and tinnitus.

Vestibular Migraine: Can overlap with Meniere's symptoms but lacks consistent auditory signs.

Signs and Diagnosis

BPPV: Positive Dix-Hallpike test; vertigo triggered by head movement.

Meniere's Disease: Vertigo with fluctuating hearing loss and worsening tinnitus.

Vestibular Neuronitis: Prolonged vertigo with associated nausea.

Vestibular Migraine: May include headache, photophobia, and phonophobia.

Investigations

Neurological examination

Pure tone audiometry

Dix-Hallpike test

Imaging (e.g., MRI) to rule out central causes like acoustic neuroma

Video head impulse testing (vHIT) to assess semicircular canal function

Treatment Strategies

BPPV: Epley maneuver (90% effective); persistent cases may require Brandt-Daroff exercises or surgery.

Vestibular Neuronitis: Symptom management with antiemetics.

Meniere's Disease: Dietary changes (low-salt), medications (betahistine, diuretics), and intratympanic injections for refractory cases.

Vestibular Migraine: Identify and avoid triggers; consider preventive medications.

Hearing Loss: Diagnosis and Management

Classification

1. Conductive Hearing Loss: Due to external or middle ear pathology.

2. Sensorineural Hearing Loss: Originates in the inner ear or auditory nerve.

Evaluation

Determine onset (sudden vs. gradual) and laterality (unilateral vs. bilateral).

Conduct pure tone audiometry and tuning fork tests (Rinne and Weber).

Management

Audiological: Hearing aids for mild-to-profound losses.

Surgical Options:

Tympanoplasty: Repairs tympanic membrane perforations.

Stapedectomy: Treats otosclerosis with prosthesis placement.

Bone-anchored hearing aids: Useful for mixed hearing loss or unilateral deafness.

Cochlear Implants: Indicated for profound sensorineural loss after multidisciplinary evaluation.

Tinnitus: Understanding and Addressing a Common Complaint

Types and Etiology

Subjective Tinnitus: Heard only by the patient; often due to noise-induced hearing loss, presbycusis, or ototoxic drugs.

Pulsatile Tinnitus: Coincides with heartbeat, typically caused by vascular abnormalities (e.g., atherosclerosis, glomus tumors).

Diagnosis

Unilateral tinnitus with hearing loss warrants MRI to exclude acoustic neuroma.

Pulsatile tinnitus may require imaging to assess vascular causes.

Management

Reassurance: Most cases are benign and self-limiting.

Masking: Noise generators or hearing aids can help.

Address underlying causes: Treat hypertension, modify medications, or manage carotid artery stenosis.

Facial Nerve Palsy: Identification and Care

Epidemiology

Bell's palsy (idiopathic) is the most common cause, with 15–40 cases per 100,000 annually.

Key Features

Symptoms: Eye dryness, drooling, and psychological impact.

Signs: Test facial nerve branches for weakness and differentiate between upper and lower motor neuron lesions.

Management

Eye Care: Prevent corneal damage with artificial tears and eyelid taping.

Medical: Oral steroids for Bell's palsy if initiated within 48 hours.

Surgical: Reserved for severe or refractory cases.

Otalgia

Description
Otalgia refers to ear pain, which may arise directly from ear-related pathology or result from referred pain originating elsewhere in the head or neck. Referred otalgia occurs due to shared neural pathways involving cranial nerves (V, VII, IX, X) and cervical nerves (C2, C3).

Epidemiology
Otalgia is a frequent complaint in primary care, particularly among children.

History and Assessment

Referred Otalgia:

Explore symptoms beyond the ear, including dental, nasal, and throat issues, to identify non-ear-related causes.

Pain referred to the ear can be caused by conditions affecting cranial nerves V (trigeminal), VII (facial), IX (glossopharyngeal), X (vagus), and upper cervical nerves (C2, C3).

Trigeminal neuralgia is the most common cause of cranial nerve-related referred otalgia.

Otorrhoea

Description
Otorrhoea involves discharge from the ear, which may consist of wax, pus, blood, mucus, or cerebrospinal fluid (CSF). Discharging wax is often normal, while other types of discharge suggest underlying pathology.

Common Pathogens

Pseudomonas aeruginosa

Staphylococcus aureus

Proteus spp.

Streptococcus pneumoniae

Haemophilus influenzae

Moraxella

History Taking

Duration of discharge (acute vs. chronic).

Associated symptoms: fever, otalgia, hearing loss, dizziness, or systemic issues.

History of trauma or foreign body insertion, particularly in children.

Use of topical antibiotics, which may predispose to fungal infections.

Consider CSF otorrhoea in cases of head trauma.

Otitis Externa

Description
Otitis is inflammation of the external auditory canal, either acute or chronic.

Epidemiology

Affects approximately 10% of people during their lifetime.

Recurrence risk increases after the initial episode.

Risk Factors

Swimming or humid climates.

Skin conditions (e.g., eczema).

Diabetes or other immunosuppression.

Trauma (e.g., excessive cleaning).

Hearing aids reduce ventilation.

Symptoms and Signs

Severe otalgia, exacerbated by pinna movement.

Itching, discharge, and possible hearing loss.

Tenderness and swelling of the external ear canal.

Complications

Peri-auricular cellulitis.

Necrotising otitis externa (a severe, potentially fatal condition causing skull base osteomyelitis).

Management

Aural toilet (e.g., microsuction).

Topical antibiotic and steroid drops (e.g., ciprofloxacin).

For necrotising otitis : hospital admission, IV antibiotics, and diabetic control.

Acute Otitis Media (AOM)

Description
Acute otitis media is an infection-driven inflammation of the middle ear, frequently seen in infants and children.

Risk Factors

Lack of breastfeeding.

Daycare attendance.

Family history of otitis media.

Age 6-18 months.

Exposure to tobacco smoke.

Symptoms

Infants: fever, irritability, vomiting.

Adults: otalgia, fever, and hearing loss.

Tympanic membrane rupture may alleviate pain but leads to discharge.

Complications

Intratemporal: tympanic membrane perforation, mastoiditis.

Intracranial: meningitis, abscesses.

Management

Analgesia (e.g., ibuprofen).

Amoxicillin for bacterial infection (10-day course).

Otitis Media with Effusion (OME)

Description
OME, or "glue ear," is characterized by a middle ear effusion without infection.

Epidemiology

Peaks at ages 2 and 5.

50% resolve within 3 months.

Symptoms

Asymptomatic or associated with hearing loss and speech delay in children.

Treatment

Observation for spontaneous resolution.

Hearing aids or surgical options (e.g., myringotomy with ventilation tube insertion).

Chronic Otitis Media

Description
Two forms:

Mucosal: Perforation of the tympanic membrane with persistent infection.

Squamous: Retraction pocket with keratin debris (cholesteatoma).

Complications
Similar to acute otitis media, with the addition of secondary otitis.

Management

Microsuction for aural toilet.

Antibiotic and steroid ear drops.

Surgical repair (e.g., myringoplasty).

Cholesteatoma

Description
Cholesteatoma is a destructive accumulation of keratinizing squamous cells in the middle ear. It is not a tumor but can erode local structures due to enzyme secretion.

Epidemiology

Occurs in both children and adults, often associated with chronic Eustachian tube dysfunction.

Management

Prompt referral to ENT for surgical intervention.

Monitoring for complications such as hearing loss and cranial nerve palsies.

Nasal Function and Anatomy: A Clinical Overview

Nasal Function

The nose primarily serves as a ventilatory organ, facilitating airflow. However, it has several additional critical roles, including:

1. Air Conditioning:

Humidification of incoming air and dehumidification of exhaled air.

Heating or cooling inspired and expired air to maintain optimal temperature for the respiratory tract.

2. Filtration:

The nasal vestibule, lined with vibrissae (small hairs), filters out large particulate matter.

3. Olfaction:

Enables the sense of smell and detection of pheromones.

4. Mucociliary Clearance:

Produces mucus that traps debris, which is transported to the pharynx via the mucociliary escalator for digestion and elimination.

5. Immune Defense:

Protects against pathogens through lysosomes, immunoglobulins (IgA, IgG), and nitric oxide production.

6. Auditory and Ocular Function:

Facilitates middle ear ventilation via the Eustachian tube.

Provides drainage for the nasolacrimal duct.

7. Resonance:

Plays a role in voice modulation and resonance.

Nasal Anatomy

The nose is divided into the external nose and the internal nasal cavity with paranasal sinuses.

1. External Nose:

Attached to the forehead by the nasal bridge, extending to a free tip.

The anterior openings, or nares, are bordered medially by the nasal septum.

The skeletal framework consists of:

Upper third: Bone (nasal bones).

Lower two-thirds: Cartilages (upper and lower lateral cartilages and septum).

Clinical Note:
The skin over the cartilaginous area contains numerous pilosebaceous glands. Pathological hypertrophy of these glands can lead to rhinophyma, characterized by an enlarged, red, bulbous nose. This condition often begins with rosacea and progresses, primarily affecting white males aged 40–60.

Internal Nasal Cavity

The nasal cavity extends from the nares to the choanae. Key features include:

1. Nasal Septum:

Composed of the maxillary crest, perpendicular plate of the ethmoid bone, and vomer. Deviations, especially anterior ones, can cause nasal obstruction.

2. Structural Components:

Roof: Formed by the sphenoid, ethmoid (cribriform plate), frontal bone, nasal bone, and cartilages.

Floor: Composed of the maxilla, palatine bone, and hard palate.

Lateral Wall: Contains turbinates (bony projections) covered by ciliated epithelium, aiding air filtration and humidification.

3. Openings in the Nasal Cavity:

Sphenoidal air cells: Drain into the spheno-ethmoidal recess.

Ethmoid sinuses: Posterior sinuses drain into the superior meatus; anterior sinuses, along with the frontal and maxillary sinuses, drain into the middle meatus.

Nasolacrimal duct: Drains into the inferior meatus.

4. Nerve Supply:

Olfactory nerve: Responsible for smell.

Trigeminal nerve: Provides general sensation via its ophthalmic and maxillary branches.

5. Blood Supply:

Derived from branches of the internal and external carotid arteries, including the anterior and posterior ethmoidal arteries, facial artery, and sphenopalatine artery.

Epistaxis (Nosebleed)

Epistaxis, though often benign, can be life-threatening. Initial assessment and management involve:

1. History:

Identifying the bleeding source (anterior vs. posterior).

Assessing frequency, volume of blood loss, and contributing factors (e.g., hypertension, anticoagulant use, trauma).

2. Management:

First-line: Lean forward, apply pressure to the soft nose, and use cold compresses for vasoconstriction.

Persistent bleeding may require identification of the bleeding site for cautery or endoscopic sphenopalatine artery ligation.

Nasal Obstruction

Common Causes:

1. Infectious: Viral, bacterial, or fungal rhinitis/rhinosinusitis.

2. Allergic: With or without nasal polyps.

3. Developmental: Septal or bony deviations.

4. Traumatic: Fractures, haematomas.

5. Iatrogenic: Surgical complications, scar tissue, or .

6. Substance Use: Chronic decongestant use or cocaine-induced vasculitis.

7. Neoplastic and Systemic Diseases: Tumors, granulomatosis, or sarcoidosis.

Fractured Nose

Key considerations in nasal trauma:

Assessment: Swelling may obscure deformities; reevaluation after 5–7 days is recommended.

Management: Manipulation under anesthesia (local or general) within the appropriate time frame.

Complications: Septal hematoma requires urgent drainage to prevent cartilage necrosis and subsequent saddle deformity.

Surgical Interventions

1. Septoplasty: Corrects deviated septum to improve nasal airflow or facilitate other procedures.

2. Septorhinoplasty: Addresses both functional and cosmetic concerns, involving cartilage and bony structures.

Chronic Rhinosinusitis (CRS)
Description
Chronic Rhinosinusitis (CRS) is a condition characterized by persistent inflammation of the nasal mucosa and paranasal sinuses lasting for more than 12 weeks. CRS can be classified into two subtypes: CRS with polyps and CRS without polyps.

Epidemiology
CRS is common and represents approximately 85% of outpatient visits related to rhinosinusitis in adults. It can often follow an episode of acute rhinosinusitis (ARS).

Causes

The etiology of CRS is multifactorial and not yet fully understood. Common contributing factors include:

Allergic causes, either intermittent or persistent.

Non-allergic causes such as occupational exposures, hormonal changes, granulomatous/inflammatory conditions, infections (viral, bacterial, fungal), anatomical abnormalities, and iatrogenic causes (e.g., medication side effects like Rhinitis Medicamentosa or cocaine abuse).

Symptoms and Signs

The diagnostic criteria for CRS, as outlined by the European Position Paper on Rhinosinusitis and Nasal Polyps (EPOS, 2012), include:

Two or more symptoms: Nasal obstruction, nasal discharge (anterior or posterior), facial pain/pressure, and a reduction or loss of smell.

Either endoscopic findings of polyps, middle meatal edema, or mucopurulent discharge, or CT findings showing mucosal changes in the ostiomeatal complex or sinuses.

Investigations

CT Sinuses: A CT scan is essential for assessing the extent of sinus disease and providing anatomical details that guide preoperative planning.

Treatment

1. Non-operative treatment:

Saline nasal irrigation to relieve symptoms.

Nasal decongestants (short course only).

Antihistamines for allergic components.

Oral steroids are used for CRS with polyps, but caution is needed due to potential side effects. Topical therapies follow oral treatment.

Topical steroids are indicated for CRS without polyps, with nasal drops like betamethasone or fluticasone typically used for 4-6 weeks, followed by maintenance with intranasal corticosteroid sprays (e.g., fluticasone or mometasone) for 3 months.

Antibiotics: The efficacy of antibiotics in CRS is still debated. According to EPOS guidelines, macrolides may be helpful in non-polyp CRS when IgE levels are normal. For CRS with polyps, doxycycline (50-100 mg/day) may be recommended.

2. Operative treatment:

Functional Endoscopic Sinus Surgery (FESS): This surgical approach aims to remove diseased tissue, alleviate obstructions, and restore sinus anatomy and function. FESS is typically considered when medical treatment fails.

Nasal Polyps
Description
Nasal polyps are benign growths that are commonly bilateral and typically present with symptoms of nasal obstruction, sometimes affecting the sense of smell. They are often associated with chronic rhinosinusitis (CRS). Types include:

Inflammatory/Allergic polyps: Grey, edematous polyps associated with CRS.

Antro-choanal polyps: A single polyp arising from the maxillary sinus, leading to unilateral nasal obstruction.

Treatment

1. Medical treatment:

A typical regimen involves a short course of oral steroids (e.g., prednisolone), followed by intranasal steroid drops for 4-6 weeks. Maintenance with intranasal corticosteroid sprays such as mometasone is common.

Antibiotics may be added if IgE levels are not elevated, with doxycycline being a commonly prescribed option.

2. Surgical treatment:

In cases where medical therapy fails, surgery is performed to remove polyps and restore sinus drainage. Functional Endoscopic Sinus Surgery (FESS) is commonly performed under general anesthesia. Risks of surgery include bleeding, infection, and recurrence of polyps.

Other Sinonasal Lesions

Benign lesions:

Papilloma/Wart: Verrucous lesions, often found in the nasal vestibule, may present with bleeding. Local excision is the typical treatment.

Pyogenic Granuloma: Friable lesions that bleed, often arising after trauma, especially in pregnancy.

Inverted Papilloma: A benign but locally aggressive lesion with a risk of recurrence and rare malignant transformation.

Juvenile Nasopharyngeal Angiofibroma (JNA): A vascular tumor affecting adolescent males, often presenting with nosebleeds and nasal obstruction. Treatment involves embolization followed by surgical removal.

Meningoencephalocoele/Glioma: A rare condition where intracranial contents herniate through a weakness in the skull base. MRI imaging is required for diagnosis.

Malignant lesions:

Sino-nasal malignancies are rare but often present late, which leads to poor prognosis. Common malignancies include squamous cell carcinoma, adenocarcinoma (often associated with woodwork exposure), and nasopharyngeal carcinoma. Treatment may include surgery, chemotherapy, or radiotherapy, depending on the type and stage.

Cleft Lip and Palate
Description
A cleft lip and/or palate is a congenital defect where there is a gap or split in the upper lip and/or roof of the mouth. This condition is the most common facial birth defect, affecting about 1 in every 700 babies. The severity can range from a minor submucous cleft to a bilateral cleft

that affects both the lip and palate, causing immediate concerns related to feeding and airway management.

Important Considerations

Feeding difficulties: Babies with a cleft lip and palate may have difficulty sucking and may experience nasal regurgitation or excessive air intake, which can lead to failure to thrive.

Otologic concerns: Children with clefts have a high incidence of middle ear issues, including glue ear, due to poor Eustachian tube function. Early hearing assessments and possible intervention (e.g., grommets) are important.

Speech and swallowing: Speech therapy is essential to address issues related to palate dysfunction and reflux.

Cosmetic issues: Surgical correction is required early in life, with possible revisions as the child grows.

Dental considerations: Dental restorations or prosthetics may be needed to support normal function and appearance.

Head and Neck Anatomy
The understanding of basic head and neck anatomy is crucial for clinical practice, especially in interpreting examination findings. Key points of interest include:

Facial Muscles: These muscles are primarily responsible for facial expressions and include the orbicularis and buccinator. They are innervated by the facial nerve and are essential for functions like chewing and speech.

Blood Supply: The external carotid artery provides the main blood supply to the face and neck, with branches including the superior thyroid artery, ascending pharyngeal artery, and lingual artery.

Conclusion

A thorough understanding of CRS, nasal polyps, and other sinonasal conditions, as well as related head and neck anatomy, is essential for accurate diagnosis and treatment planning. Proper clinical examination, investigations, and patient management, including both medical and surgical interventions, are key to improving patient outcomes.

Topographic Anatomy of the Neck

The anatomical regions of the neck are systematically categorized into levels, designated by Roman numerals. This classification is particularly advantageous when pinpointing the location of a neck mass. Although these levels can be further subdivided, such details are beyond the scope of this handbook.

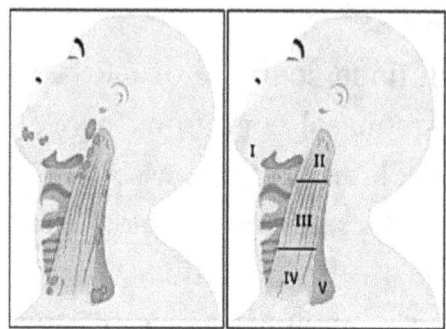

Fig. 15: Levels of the Neck

The neck can also be anatomically divided into two major triangles: the anterior and posterior triangles.

Anterior Triangle:
This area is delineated by the following boundaries:

Superiorly: The mandible.

Laterally: The sternocleidomastoid muscle.

Medially: The midline of the neck.

Posterior Triangle:
The boundaries of this region include:

Anteromedially: The sternocleidomastoid muscle.

Inferiorly: The clavicle.

Posteriorly: The trapezius muscle.

Detailed Overview of Neck Anatomy, Clinical Assessment, and Associated Pathologies

Fascial Layers of the Neck

Superficial Layer: A thin sheet of fascia encasing the platysma muscle.

Deep Fascia: Divided into three distinct layers:

1. Investing Layer (External): Encloses the trapezius, sternocleidomastoid, and parotid

gland. The deeper portion forms the carotid sheath, housing critical vascular structures

2. Pretracheal Layer (Visceral): Covers the salivary glands, thyroid, and other anterior tracheal structures

3. Prevertebral Layer (Internal): Surrounds the prevertebral muscles, with the retropharyngeal space lying between this layer and the pharynx (Figure 56).

Swallowing Physiology

1. Oral Phase (Voluntary):

Preparatory: Food bolus is formed and secured anteriorly; the soft palate and tongue close the posterior oral cavity to prevent leakage.

Propulsive: The tongue's dorsum pushes the bolus posteriorly into the oropharynx.

2. Pharyngeal Phase (Involuntary, CN IX):

The soft palate elevates, sealing the nasopharynx to prevent nasal regurgitation.

The larynx elevates and closes to protect the airway, while pharyngeal constrictor muscles propel the bolus downward.

3. Esophageal Phase:

The upper esophageal sphincter (UES) relaxes to allow bolus entry.

Peristalsis, aided by gravity in an upright posture, moves the bolus toward the lower esophageal sphincter (LES).

History-Taking for a Neck Lump

1. Opening Questions:

"What is your age and occupation?"

"What brought you here today?"

2. History of Presenting Complaint:

"When did you first notice the lump?"

"Has it changed in size or consistency?"

"Is it always present or intermittent?"

"Have you experienced pain, difficulty swallowing, or breathing issues?"

"Have you noticed any associated symptoms, such as weight loss, fever, or night sweats?"

3. Past Medical History:

Previous investigations or treatments for the lump.

4. Social History:

Smoking and alcohol consumption, with quantification.

5. Red Flag Symptoms:

Persistent or enlarging lumps (3–6 weeks).

Hoarseness lasting over three weeks.

Dysphagia or unexplained sore throat.

Common Causes of Neck Lumps

By Age:

Children/Young Adults: Inflammatory > Congenital > Neoplastic.

Adults: Inflammatory > Neoplastic > Congenital.

Older Adults: Neoplastic > Inflammatory.

Branchial Cysts

Description:

Typically present in young adults as upper neck masses. These epithelial inclusions within lymph nodes can become infected. In older adults, such cysts warrant investigation for potential malignancy.

Investigations:

Ultrasound and fine needle aspiration cytology (FNAC), supplemented by cross-sectional imaging.

Treatment:

Surgical excision.

Dysphagia (Difficulty Swallowing)

History:

Establish the level (pharynx, esophagus) and type (solids, liquids).

Assess for associated symptoms: hoarseness, painful swallowing, regurgitation, weight loss.

Screen for cancer risk factors (e.g., smoking, alcohol).

Causes:

Extraluminal: Neck masses, vascular anomalies, mediastinal masses.

Intramural: Neurological or muscular disorders (e.g., CVA, achalasia).

Intraluminal: Foreign bodies, strictures, malignancies.

Investigations:

Blood tests, imaging (CT/MRI), barium swallow, and dynamic studies like video fluoroscopy.

Dysphonia (Hoarseness)

Description:

A disorder affecting vocal quality, pitch, or loudness.

Causes:

Malignant: Squamous cell carcinoma.

Benign: Vocal cord nodules, cysts.

Neuromuscular: Vocal cord palsy.

Infective: Laryngitis, fungal infections.

Iatrogenic: Post-surgical complications, such as recurrent laryngeal nerve injury.

Investigations:

Flexible nasendoscopy and relevant blood tests.

Red Flags:

Persistent hoarseness, neck mass, unexplained weight loss, or neurological symptoms.

Management of Urgent ENT Symptoms

Persistent hoarseness or dysphagia.

Rapidly enlarging neck lumps.

Associated systemic symptoms such as fever, unexplained weight loss, or persistent sore throat.

Tonsillitis Overview

Definition:
Tonsillitis refers to inflammation and infection of the palatine tonsils. It can be caused by viral or bacterial pathogens, with varying clinical presentations and severity.

Epidemiology

Prevalence: Commonly affects children and young adults.

Etiology:

Viral Causes (70%): Majority of cases are viral, reducing the effectiveness of antibiotic treatment.

Bacterial Causes (30%): Most frequently caused by Group A beta-hemolytic streptococci (GABHS).

Other bacterial agents include:

Haemophilus influenzae

Streptococcus pneumoniae

Staphylococcus species (associated with dehydration and prior antibiotic use).

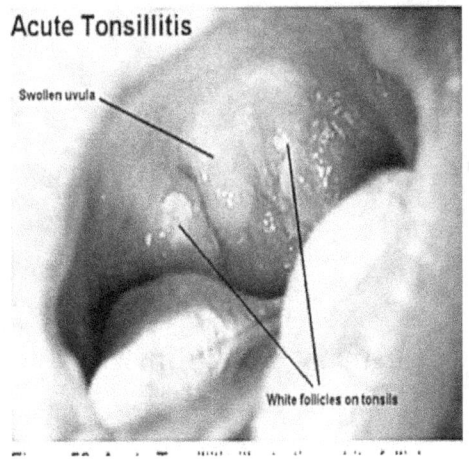

Fig. 16: White Follicles on Inflamed Tonsils

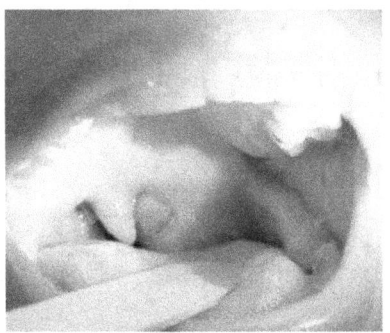

Fig. 17: Left-Sided Peritonsillar Abscess (Quinsy)

Symptoms

General:

Sore throat (primary complaint).

Odynophagia (pain during swallowing) or dysphagia (difficulty swallowing).

Ear pain (referred otalgia).

Systemic symptoms such as malaise and headache.

Specific to Viral Tonsillitis: Typically presents with less severe symptoms.

Clinical Signs

Fever: Elevated body temperature.

Tonsillar Findings:

Enlarged, swollen tonsils.

Presence of exudates (white spots or patches).

Thickened or "hot potato" voice.

Additional Findings:

Trismus: Difficulty opening the mouth, suggestive of a peritonsillar abscess (quinsy).

Cervical Lymphadenopathy: Swollen and tender lymph nodes on both sides of the neck.

Visual Representation

Figure 58 demonstrates acute tonsillitis with visible white follicles on the tonsils. (Image reference courtesy of Otolaryngology Houston).

Clinical Notes:

Early differentiation between viral and bacterial tonsillitis is crucial for management. Viral cases usually resolve with supportive care, while bacterial infections may require antibiotic treatment to prevent complications such as peritonsillar abscesses or rheumatic fever.

Pharyngeal Pouch (Zenker's Diverticulum)

Overview:
Zenker's diverticulum refers to an outpouching of the pharyngeal mucosa and submucosa. It develops in the posterior pharyngeal wall, specifically at Killian's dehiscence—a region of weakness between the cricopharyngeus and thyropharyngeus muscles of the upper esophageal sphincter.

Epidemiology:

Predominantly affects elderly males.

Rare condition, with an incidence of approximately 2 cases per 100,000 annually in the UK.

Pathophysiology:
The exact cause remains unclear, but a leading theory suggests a lack of coordination between the cricopharyngeus muscle's relaxation and peristaltic movements, hindering bolus passage through the hypopharynx.

Clinical Features:

Asymptomatic in early stages or if small.

Progressive Symptoms: Dysphagia, sensation of a lump in the throat, regurgitation of undigested food, halitosis due to food stasis in the pouch, and recurrent chest infections caused by aspiration.

Signs:

Audible gurgling sounds and persistent bad breath.

Normal findings on ENT examinations are common.

Diagnostics:

Gold Standard: Barium swallow imaging confirms the diagnosis.

Supplementary Test: Rigid esophagoscopy to rule out malignancy within the pouch.

Management:

Asymptomatic Cases: Conservative observation.

Symptomatic Cases: Endoscopic stapling is the preferred approach. For patients unsuitable for endoscopy, open surgical techniques with cricopharyngeal muscle division are considered.

Globus Pharyngeus

Overview:
A subjective sensation of a lump or foreign body in the throat without any structural or pathological findings. It is typically linked to stress, anxiety, or laryngopharyngeal reflux.

Epidemiology:
Frequently encountered in ENT clinics, often attributed to psychological or functional causes.

Diagnostic Workup:

Comprehensive ENT evaluation with flexible nasopharyngolaryngoscopy to exclude organic pathology.

In patients with risk factors like smoking or excessive alcohol intake, additional tests (e.g., barium swallow, CT scan, or upper GI endoscopy) are necessary to evaluate for malignancy.

Management:

Reassurance and lifestyle modifications are the cornerstone of treatment.

Optimal anti-reflux therapy is recommended for symptom control.

Thyroid Masses

Overview:
Thyroid masses are the most common presentations of thyroid-related conditions, often causing compressive symptoms such as difficulty swallowing (dysphagia) or breathing (dyspnea).

Diagnostic Steps:

1. Imaging:

Neck ultrasound is the first-line modality to evaluate and stratify thyroid lesions.

It assesses malignancy risk, presence of lymphadenopathy, and determines whether the lesion is solitary or part of a multinodular goiter.

2. Fine Needle Aspiration Cytology (FNAC):

FNAC is essential for evaluating suspicious nodules, especially for diagnosing papillary thyroid carcinoma.

Limitations: FNAC cannot differentiate between follicular adenoma and carcinoma due to the need for histopathological assessment of capsular or vascular invasion.

3. Additional Tests:

Thyroid function tests to assess hormonal activity.

Advanced imaging (e.g., CT) may be warranted for retrosternal goiters.

Management:

Non-Surgical: Observation and medical therapy (e.g., antithyroid drugs for hyperthyroidism).

Surgical Indications: Significant mass effect, suspicion of malignancy, or uncontrolled symptoms. Post-thyroidectomy, patients may require thyroid hormone replacement therapy.

Thyroid Cancer

Epidemiology and Risk Factors:

Incidence in the UK: ~3.4 cases per 100,000 annually, with a mortality rate of ~0.4 per 100,000.

More prevalent in women; risk factors include radiation exposure and familial predisposition.

Classification and Staging:

Papillary and follicular types are most common, followed by medullary and anaplastic thyroid cancers.

Ultrasound is the primary staging tool, supplemented by non-contrast CT or MRI for selected cases.

Management:

1. Surgical Options:

Lobectomy for small, low-risk lesions (<1 cm).

Total thyroidectomy for larger or high-risk malignancies (>1 cm).

Neck dissection may be necessary for metastatic lymphadenopathy.

2. Adjuvant Therapy:

Postoperative radioiodine ablation (RAI) is tailored based on risk stratification, with proven survival benefits in differentiated cancers.

Levothyroxine suppresses TSH, reducing recurrence risk.

3. Follow-Up:

Regular monitoring with thyroglobulin levels (tumor marker) and periodic ultrasound.

Medullary Thyroid Carcinoma (MTC)

Pathophysiology:

Arises from parafollicular C-cells, with 80% sporadic cases and 20% familial associations (e.g., MEN 2 syndromes).

Diagnostic Approach:

Neck ultrasound, FNAC, and tumor marker evaluation (calcitonin, CEA).

Genetic screening for RET proto-oncogene mutations.

Management:

Total thyroidectomy with neck dissection.

Prophylactic surgery may be considered for high-risk familial cases.

RAI therapy is ineffective due to the absence of iodine uptake.

Anaplastic Thyroid Cancer

Clinical Features:
A rare, aggressive malignancy presenting as a rapidly enlarging neck mass, often with poor prognosis.

Diagnostic and Therapeutic Strategy:

Core or open biopsy is essential for confirmation.

Management is primarily palliative, focusing on symptom relief.

Thyroid Lymphoma

Epidemiology and Risk Factor:

Rare malignancy linked to Hashimoto's thyroiditis.

Presents as a rapidly growing goiter with compressive symptoms.

Diagnostics and Treatment:

Diagnosis relies on core or open biopsy.

Management follows standard lymphoma protocols with chemotherapy and radiotherapy.

Carcinoma of the Oropharynx

Definition
Oropharyngeal carcinoma primarily involves tumors originating from the posterior third of the tongue and the tonsils (or tonsillar fossae in patients who have undergone tonsillectomy). Approximately 70% of tonsillar carcinomas are squamous cell carcinoma (SCC), with a minority being lymphomas.

Risk Factors

Tobacco Use: Long-standing smoking history significantly increases risk.

Alcohol Consumption: Synergistic effect with smoking.

Human Papillomavirus (HPV): Strong association, particularly with subtypes HPV 16 and 18.

Emerging Trends: Rising incidence in younger adults, especially non-smokers, due to HPV-related carcinomas.

Clinical Presentation

Unilateral, painless tonsillar swelling.

Throat discomfort progressing to dysphagia.

Referred ear pain (Arnold's nerve involvement).

Sensation of a lump in the throat.

Metastatic cervical lymphadenopathy, particularly jugulodigastric nodes.

Trismus (a concerning sign of local tissue invasion).

Diagnostic Approach

1. Comprehensive head and neck examination.

2. Panendoscopy with biopsy of suspicious lesions.

3. Fine needle aspiration (FNA) for palpable neck lymph nodes.

4. Imaging:

MRI: For detailed tumor delineation.

CT Scans: Staging of neck, chest, and abdomen.

Management

Localized Disease: Surgical excision with or without adjuvant radiotherapy.

Advanced Disease: Combined chemoradiotherapy.

Carcinoma of the Hypopharynx

Definition
Hypopharyngeal carcinomas most frequently arise in the pyriform sinus. Nearly all are squamous cell carcinomas, known for early and extensive metastatic spread. The disease predominantly affects males aged 55–70 with significant tobacco and/or alcohol use.

Symptoms

Cervical lymphadenopathy.

Radiating throat pain, often extending to the ear.

Progressive dysphagia or odynophagia.

Voice changes.

Paterson-Brown-Kelly Syndrome: Dysphagia, hypochromic microcytic anemia, esophageal webs, and potential postcricoid carcinoma development.

Investigations

1. Endoscopy with biopsy confirmation.

2. Pharyngo-oesophagoscopy to assess the extent of involvement.

3. Imaging:

Barium swallow for functional assessment.

MRI and staging CT for disease extent.

Treatment Options

Early Disease: Surgery with or without adjuvant radiotherapy (rare).

Advanced Disease: Multimodal therapy including surgery, radiotherapy, and potential neoadjuvant chemotherapy.

Incurable Cases: Palliative care focused on symptom relief.

Carcinoma of the Larynx

Definition
Laryngeal cancer is categorized into three regions:

1. Supraglottis: Extends from the epiglottis to the laryngeal ventricle.

2. Glottis: Includes true vocal folds and extends 1 cm inferiorly.

3. Subglottis: Below the glottis to the cricoid cartilage.

The most common histological subtype is SCC, representing 90% of cases.

Epidemiology

Male predominance, especially in older adults.

In younger populations, the male-to-female ratio is closer to 1:1.

Risk Factors

Tobacco use (primary contributor).

Alcohol consumption (cumulative risk increases with smoking).

Symptoms

Glottic Cancer: Hoarseness, progressively worsening over weeks to months.

Supraglottic Cancer: Noisy breathing, stridor, and dysphagia.

Late-stage presentations may include cough, hemoptysis, and neck lymphadenopathy.

Investigations

ENT examination, including flexible nasoendoscopy.

Microlaryngoscopy with biopsy.

Staging with CT or MRI, and occasionally PET CT.

Management

Early Disease (T1, T2): Radiotherapy or endoscopic laser excision.

Advanced Disease (T3, T4): Multimodal approaches including chemoradiotherapy or laryngectomy with postoperative radiotherapy.

Laryngopharyngeal Reflux (LPR)

Definition
LPR encompasses upper respiratory symptoms caused by gastric content irritation of the larynx.

Symptoms

Hoarseness, throat clearing, chronic cough.

Globus sensation and dysphagia.

Minimal correlation with classic gastroesophageal reflux symptoms like heartburn.

Diagnosis

Reflux Symptom Index (RSI): Scores >13 indicate LPR.

Laryngoscopic Findings: Edema, erythema, thick mucus, or granulomas.

Objective Measures: 24-hour dual-probe pH monitoring remains the gold standard.

Management

1. Lifestyle Modifications:

Avoid meals before bedtime.

Reduce smoking and alcohol consumption.

Address obesity and dietary habits.

2. Pharmacotherapy:

Alginate-based formulations.

Proton pump inhibitors (PPIs) with limited evidence.

3. Refractory Cases: Referral to gastroenterologists for further evaluation.

Snoring and Obstructive Sleep Apnea (OSA)

Definition
OSA involves episodic airway obstruction during sleep, leading to apneas (breath-holding >10 seconds) or hypopneas (reduced airflow with oxygen desaturation).

Epidemiology

Affects 1–4% of adults, predominantly males.

Classified by Apnea-Hypopnea Index (AHI):

Mild: 5–15.

Moderate: 16–30.

Severe: >30.

Symptoms

Witnessed apneas, choking, or gasping during sleep.

Daytime fatigue and irritability.

Snoring with restlessness.

Diagnosis

Detailed history and ENT examination.

Polysomnography (gold standard).

Epworth Sleepiness Score for daytime somnolence (>10 is abnormal).

Treatment

1. Lifestyle Modifications:

Weight loss.

Avoid alcohol and supine sleep positions.

2. Devices:

CPAP for airway splinting.

Mandibular advancement devices.

3. Surgery: Reserved for refractory cases and tailored to anatomical causes.

Children: Adenotonsillectomy is effective.

Adults: May involve palatal surgery, tonsillectomy, or septoplasty, but evidence for effectiveness is limited.

Acute Airway Obstruction

Overview
Acute airway obstruction represents a critical medical emergency that requires immediate recognition and management to prevent fatal outcomes.

Etiology

Adults

Infectious Causes: Conditions such as deep neck space infections.

Neoplastic Causes: Head and neck malignancies, including tumors of the tongue base, oropharynx, or larynx.

Children

Infectious Causes: Common examples include croup and epiglottitis.

Foreign Bodies: Frequently implicated, especially in younger children.

Congenital Conditions: Laryngomalacia and subglottic stenosis are notable examples.

Clinical Presentation

Symptoms:

Shortness of breath and noisy breathing (commonly stridor).

Voice alterations.

Cough.

Stridor Classification:

Inspiratory: Obstruction above the glottis.

Expiratory: Obstruction below the carina.

Biphasic: Obstruction at the glottis or subglottic level.

Signs:

Tachypnea.

Use of accessory muscles.

Cyanosis or agitation.

Audible breathing abnormalities, such as stertor or stridor.

Decreased breath sounds, indicating fatigue or acute decompensation.

Complications

Respiratory arrest due to unrecognized or unaddressed airway compromise.

Children are at a heightened risk for rapid deterioration.

Investigations

Diagnostic evaluation is secondary to stabilizing the airway.

Imaging should be avoided in unstable patients.

Nasendoscopy can be performed in stable cases to identify the cause.

Management

1. General Measures:

Seek early involvement of senior specialists (ENT, anesthesiology, pediatrics).

Administer oxygen or Heliox (a mixture of helium and oxygen) to enhance airflow.

2. Medications:

Nebulized Adrenaline: 1 mL of 1:1000 adrenaline diluted in 4 mL saline.

Steroids: Dexamethasone (0.1–0.2 mg/kg IV or nebulized).

3. Advanced Interventions:

Intubation: Fiberoptic intubation may be utilized to secure the airway.

Nasopharyngeal Airway: Useful in cases of upper airway swelling (e.g., angioedema).

Tracheostomy or Cricothyroidotomy: Emergency procedures to bypass airway obstructions.

Epistaxis (Nosebleed)

Overview
Epistaxis is one of the most common ENT emergencies, categorized as anterior or posterior bleeding based on its origin.

History

Timing, triggers (e.g., trauma), and the volume of bleeding.

Unilateral vs. bilateral bleeding and whether blood is swallowed (suggesting posterior bleeding).

Assess systemic risk factors such as coagulopathy or hypertension.

Causes

Local: Trauma, infections, or nasal sprays.

Systemic: Coagulopathies, pregnancy, substance abuse, and hypertension.

Management

1. Initial Measures:

Direct pressure over Little's area for 10 minutes.

Chemical cauterization with silver nitrate sticks for localized bleeding (avoid bilateral application).

2. Persistent Bleeding:

Anterior nasal packing with appropriate materials.

Posterior nasal packing, often using a Foley catheter.

3. Severe Cases:

Surgical intervention, such as arterial ligation or interventional radiology embolization, may be required.

Foreign Body in the Nose

Overview

Common in children, nasal foreign bodies can lead to obstruction or complications if aspirated.

Presentation

Unilateral, often offensive nasal discharge.

Nasal obstruction or irritability.

Management

Removal techniques include positive pressure or the use of specialized instruments such as an earwax hook or alligator forceps.

General anesthesia may be required in complex cases.

Nasal Septal Hematoma

Overview

A nasal septal hematoma results from trauma and requires prompt intervention to avoid complications such as cartilage necrosis or saddle-nose deformity.

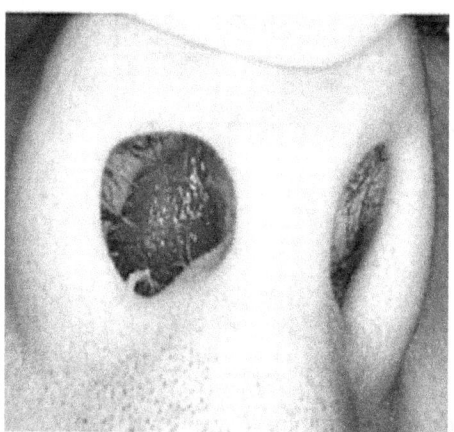

Fig. 18: Right-Sided Septal Hematoma: Blood Accumulation Between the Perichondrium and Septal Cartilage

Management

Urgent incision and drainage under general anesthesia.

Antibiotic therapy to prevent infection.

Foreign Body in the Ear

Overview
Foreign bodies in the ear are frequently observed in children but can occur in adults due to accidents (e.g., cotton bud fragments).

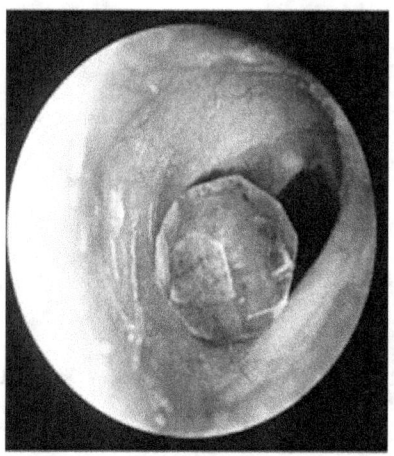

Fig. 19: Central Perforation of Left Tympanic Membrane

Management

Removal depends on the object type and location, employing tools like wax hooks or alligator forceps.

Avoid further pushing the foreign object.

Perforated Tympanic Membrane

Causes: Trauma, infections (e.g., otitis media), or previous surgeries.
Management:

Advise patients to avoid water exposure.

Traumatic perforations often heal within 6–8 weeks.

Antibiotic drops may be needed for infected perforations.

Surgical repair (myringoplasty) for recurrent or non-healing cases.

Foreign Body in the Pharynx or Esophagus

Causes

Children: Commonly involves ingestion of inanimate objects like coins. A high index of suspicion for button batteries is essential as they may resemble coins on X-rays but pose a greater risk due to chemical burns, potentially leading to esophageal perforation within hours.

Adults: Often involves food boluses. Identifying whether a bone is present is critical, as this significantly increases the risk of esophageal perforation and requires urgent intervention.

Presentation

General Symptoms: Dysphagia (difficulty swallowing), odynophagia (painful swallowing), and drooling.

Children: Symptoms may be nonspecific, such as refusal to eat or lethargy.

Management

Batteries: Immediate removal is a surgical emergency, akin to managing an airway obstruction or significant bleed.

Food Bolus with Bone: Requires prompt removal to prevent esophageal perforation.

Food Bolus without Bone: May pass spontaneously during sleep due to muscle relaxation or with the administration of muscle relaxants like hyoscine butylbromide (Buscopan). If the bolus does not pass, further interventions such as rigid esophagoscopy or OGD (esophagogastroduodenoscopy) may be necessary. A water swallow test can help localize the obstruction: immediate regurgitation suggests high obstruction, while delayed regurgitation indicates low obstruction.

Deep Neck Space Infections

Causes

Typically bacterial in origin, often due to poor dental hygiene. Ludwig's angina is a notable example, usually arising from dental infections.

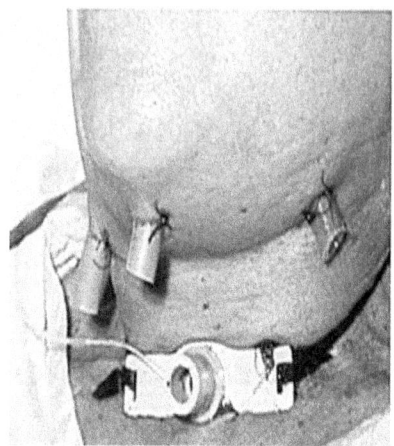

Fig. 20: Ludwig's Angina

Presentation

Symptoms vary based on the affected deep neck space but commonly include:

Pain, dysphagia, dysphonia (altered voice), drooling, trismus (difficulty opening the mouth), and stridor.

Systemic signs: Pyrexia, malaise, and a generally unwell appearance.

Children: Retropharyngeal infections are more common, presenting with swallowing difficulties, trismus, limited neck movement, or torticollis (twisted neck posture).

Adults: Parapharyngeal infections are more prevalent. Nasendoscopy may reveal a parapharyngeal bulge.

Management

1. Initial Approach:

Apply the "ABC" protocol (Airway, Breathing, Circulation) due to the high risk of airway compromise, which may require intubation or tracheostomy.

2. Medical Management:

Intravenous fluids and broad-spectrum antibiotics such as co-amoxiclav.

Contrast-enhanced CT imaging to identify the affected spaces and confirm the diagnosis.

3. Definitive Treatment:

Surgical drainage of abscesses via peroral or external approaches, depending on the location.

Small collections (<1 cm) may respond to antibiotics alone.

Microbiological culture results from pus or blood samples guide targeted therapy.

Special Considerations

Quinsy (Peritonsillar Abscess):

Symptoms include severe pain, odynophagia, trismus, and a "hot-potato" voice.

Treated with peroral aspiration or incision and drainage under local anesthesia.

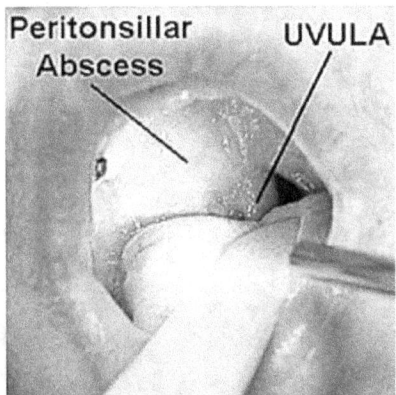

Fig. 21: Right quin

Ludwig's Angina:

Rapidly spreading infection of the floor of the mouth and submandibular space, often due to dental sources.

Requires surgical drainage and elimination of the infection source, such as extracting a decayed tooth.

Penetrating Neck Trauma: Causes, Presentation, and Management

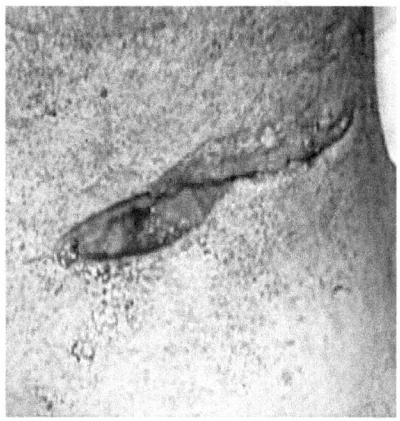

Fig. 22: Neck Laceration by Knife

Causes

Penetrating neck injuries commonly result from sharp objects such as knives, broken glass (e.g., bottles used as weapons), or gunshot wounds. These injuries often involve critical anatomical structures, posing significant risks to vascular, respiratory, and neurological systems.

Presentation

A thorough history is crucial, including details about the mechanism of injury (e.g., type of weapon, time since injury, and depth of penetration). Examination should focus on the wound's location, which provides clues to the affected structures. The neck is anatomically divided into three zones:

Zone I: Extends from the clavicle to the cricoid cartilage. Key structures include the common carotid artery, internal jugular vein, trachea, and esophagus.

Zone II: Ranges from the cricoid cartilage to the angle of the mandible. This is the most frequently injured zone, containing the larynx, pharynx, carotid artery bifurcation, internal jugular vein, and cranial nerves (e.g., vagus, hypoglossal, and spinal accessory nerves).

Zone III: Stretches from the angle of the mandible to the skull base, involving structures like the internal carotid artery, cranial nerves, and skull base.

Management

The Advanced Trauma Life Support (ATLS) protocol is the cornerstone of managing penetrating neck trauma:

1. Airway (A): Ensure a secure airway via intubation or surgical methods (e.g., cricothyroidotomy, tracheostomy) if compromised.

2. Breathing (B): Monitor and manage respiratory function.

3. Circulation (C): Assess for active bleeding or vascular compromise, with hemostasis prioritized.

4. Disability (D): Evaluate neurological status for cranial nerve or spinal cord involvement.

5. Exposure (E): Inspect all potential injury sites for additional wounds or complications.

Imaging: In hemodynamically stable patients, advanced imaging such as CT angiography can identify vascular injuries or assess for damage to the spine, esophagus, or trachea.

Surgical Exploration: If the platysma muscle is breached, surgical intervention is generally required. However, in stable patients without immediate complications, conservative management with imaging and observation is increasingly considered safe and effective.

Early identification and precise management are critical to minimizing morbidity and mortality in penetrating neck trauma cases.

Antibiotic and Steroid Use in ENT: A Detailed Overview

Antibiotics

Antibiotics in ENT practice are administered topically (e.g., ear drops), orally, or intravenously, depending on the condition and severity. Commonly used antibiotics include:

1. Phenoxymethylpenicillin

Indication: Effective for bacterial sore throats, including tonsillitis.

Duration: Typically prescribed for 10 days.

2. Amoxicillin

Indication: Treats sinusitis and otitis media caused by bacterial infections.

Precaution: Should not be used for sore throats if glandular fever is suspected, as it may cause severe skin reactions or Stevens-Johnson syndrome.

3. Flucloxacillin

Indication: Used for staphylococcal infections, including cellulitis.

4. Macrolides (e.g., erythromycin, clarithromycin)

Indication: Alternative for patients allergic to penicillin; used for bacterial infections and chronic rhinosinusitis without polyposis.

5. Aminoglycosides (e.g., gentamicin combined with steroids)

Indication: Treats otitis caused by Pseudomonas (an opportunistic pathogen).

Precaution: Use cautiously with perforated tympanic membranes or grommets due to ototoxicity risks.

6. Quinolones (e.g., ciprofloxacin)

Indication: Treats pseudomonas otitis and chronic suppurative otitis media with a perforated tympanic membrane.

Note: Ciprofloxacin ear drops are unlicensed in the UK but frequently used in eye-drop form due to lower ototoxicity risks.

Antifungals

Clotrimazole: Effective for fungal otitis, particularly Candida infections.

Steroids

1. Topical Nasal Steroids

Indication: Used for allergic rhinitis and chronic rhinosinusitis (with or without polyposis).

Examples:

Fluticasone spray/nasules

Mometasone spray

Beclomethasone spray/nasules

Notes:

Minimal systemic absorption.

Common side effects: nasal dryness, crusting, and irritation, which can be mitigated by applying petroleum jelly.

Improvement may take 2–3 weeks, with reevaluation recommended if no improvement occurs after 8 weeks.

2. Oral Steroids

Indication: Prescribed in conditions such as:

Nasal polyposis: Used alongside topical steroids.

Bell's Palsy: Early administration (within 24–48 hours) improves nerve recovery.

Sudden Sensorineural Hearing Loss: Traditionally treated with oral steroids, though intratympanic dexamethasone is gaining preference due to better evidence of efficacy.

Antihistamines

Indication: Effective for rhinitis symptoms like sneezing, rhinorrhea, and eye itching.

Usage: Often combined with or used alongside topical corticosteroids.

Side Effects: Systemic antihistamines may cause sedation, dry mouth, blurry vision, urinary retention, and acute angle glaucoma.

Vestibular Sedatives and Meniere's Disease

1. Prochlorperazine

Indication: Prescribed for nausea and vertigo caused by labyrinthitis.

Precaution: Should not be used for longer than two weeks to allow natural brain compensation.

2. Cinnarizine

Indication: Treats nausea and vertigo; also an antihistamine and calcium antagonist.

3. Betahistine

Indication: Traditionally used for Meniere's disease, although evidence for efficacy is limited. Believed to reduce endolymphatic pressure by improving blood flow to the inner ear.

4. Intratympanic Injections (Dexamethasone or Gentamicin)

Indication: Used for Meniere's disease.

Notes:

Dexamethasone is preferred for patients with good hearing due to its non-ototoxic nature.

Gentamicin, though ototoxic, is used in cases of severe disease to reduce vestibular nerve function.

Practical Procedures in ENT

Nasal Cautery

Silver nitrate cautery of the anterior nasal septum is a fundamental skill for junior ENT doctors. To perform the procedure effectively, universal precautions should be observed, and essential tools like a headlight and suction (such as Zollner or Fraser) are required.

Start by decongesting and numbing the nasal passages using a combination of lignocaine and phenylephrine, either by spraying directly into the nose or applying it with cotton pledgets. A careful examination of the anterior septum will often reveal the source of the bleeding, such as in the right Little's area (Figure 74). The vasoconstrictive effect of the local anesthetic helps to slow down any active bleeding, allowing for easier cautery.

Silver nitrate should be applied in a "rose-petal" pattern (Figure 76), ensuring that the cautery is focused on the bleeding site without overextending. After cauterization, Naseptin cream (a combination of Chlorhexidine and Neomycin) can be applied for up to two weeks to aid healing. However, caution is required when using this cream, as it contains Arachis oil, which can cause an allergic reaction in individuals with a peanut allergy. It's also essential not to cauterize both sides of the septum directly opposite each other, as this could lead to a septal perforation. Some institutions may use bipolar cautery, but the fundamental principles of cauterization remain consistent.

Anterior Nasal Packing

If cautery is unsuccessful in identifying or controlling the bleeding, anterior nasal packing may be necessary. Nasal packs are generally categorized into anterior or posterior. Common anterior packing options include Merocel nasal tampons, which support clot stabilization, and Rapid Rhino packs, which provide both clot support and internal balloon pressure to help stop bleeding.

As with cautery, it is important to use universal precautions, a headlight, suction, and an assistant. Properly anesthetize the nose as described earlier. Inform the patient of the procedure and advise them that some discomfort may occur during insertion.

The pack should be carefully inserted along the floor of the nasal cavity, between the septum and the inferior turbinate (Figure 77). Anatomical variations, such as septal deviations, may make this procedure more challenging. If the source of bleeding is unclear or unilateral packing does not control the hemorrhage, bilateral packing may be necessary, though this can exacerbate cardiopulmonary issues.

Ensure that the patient is adequately anesthetized to tolerate the packing, and prescribe appropriate analgesia. Once inserted, the patient should be closely monitored, and clotting abnormalities should be managed with input from specialists, such as hematology or cardiology. After 15 minutes, re-examine the patient to assess the effectiveness of the packing. If bleeding persists or a posterior bleed is suspected, posterior nasal packing may be required. This should ideally be done under senior supervision. The traditional method involves a Foley urinary catheter with a balloon to occlude the posterior nasal space, although newer options like the Antero-Posterior Rapid Rhino and Brighton Epistaxis Balloons are now available.

Nasendoscopy

Nasendoscopy, which uses a flexible fiberoptic endoscope or a rigid scope, allows for examination of the nose, pharynx, and larynx. This procedure can be done in the outpatient setting, often without the need for anesthesia.

Indications:

Assessing the nose, sinuses, pharynx, and larynx for pathology

Evaluating the voice

Investigating swallowing issues

Assessing the airway, particularly during intubation

Technique: The endoscope should be accompanied by a high-quality light source, with the image viewable either through an eyepiece or on a screen. This method facilitates teaching, allows the patient to view the procedure, and enables recording of images or videos. Portable, battery-operated endoscopes are available for use in various settings, including wards.

While some patients may require local anesthesia (such as a lidocaine/phenylephrine spray), many tolerate the procedure without it. The patient should be seated upright, with slight flexion of the head. Position the screen at an appropriate distance to maintain a clear view of the endoscope's image. Ensure the tip of the endoscope is clean for optimal visibility.

The examination involves inspecting the nasal turbinates, septum, and mucosa, as well as assessing for any mucus, pus, or polyps. Other structures to examine include the nasopharynx, posterior pharyngeal wall, soft palate, uvula, tonsillar region, tongue base, epiglottis, vocal folds, and their mobility by asking the patient to say "eeeeeeeee."

The procedure typically takes under two minutes. It is important to warn the patient to refrain from eating or drinking for 30 minutes if a local anesthetic has been used.

Oto-Microscopy and Foreign Body Removal

Examination of the ear under a microscope is often performed by ENT specialists due to the need for specific equipment.

Indications:

Examining the ear

Removing impacted ear wax

Treating ear infections

Removing foreign bodies

Technique: The patient should lie on their back on an exam table. Elevating the head may be necessary for patients who experience difficulty breathing when lying flat. The clinician should adjust the microscope for comfort and clear visualization, ensuring proper focus before beginning the procedure.

Equipment required may include suction, a wax hook, Jobson-Horne probe, crocodile forceps, and an aural speculum. Foreign body removal is usually most successful on the first attempt, particularly in children. If the initial attempt fails, general anesthesia may be necessary.

For soft foreign bodies like cotton wool, crocodile forceps are effective. Hard objects, such as beads, are best removed using a wax hook or Jobson-Horne probe. If an insect is present, especially if alive, it should first be immobilized with olive oil.

By following these techniques and guidelines, ENT practitioners can effectively manage a range of common conditions such as epistaxis, foreign body removal, and nasal and ear assessments, ensuring improved patient outcomes.

Comprehensive Overview of Audiological Assessments

Pure Tone Audiometry (PTA)

Definition

Pure Tone Audiometry (PTA) evaluates an individual's hearing threshold by determining the quietest sounds they can detect at various frequencies. This subjective test relies on the patient's responses to auditory stimuli, typically measured in decibels (dB) using a logarithmic scale. Common sound intensity references include:

Whisper at 1 meter: 30 dB

Normal conversation: 60 dB

Shouting: 90 dB

Discomfort threshold: ~120 dB

Procedure

1. Equipment and Setup:
An audiometer generates pure tone sounds at variable frequencies. Testing is conducted in a soundproof room to ensure accuracy, with the subject unable to observe adjustments being made to the audiometer.

2. Pre-Test Examination:

Ensure the absence of ear canal blockages, infections, or wax accumulation.

Use headphones for air conduction testing, followed by a bone vibrator on the mastoid process for bone conduction testing.

3. Testing Frequencies:

Air conduction: 250–8000 Hz

Bone conduction: 500–4000 Hz

4. Masking Techniques:
To prevent crossover hearing (detection by the non-test ear), masking noise is introduced to the opposite ear.

Interpretation of Results

Hearing thresholds are categorized as follows:

Normal hearing: ≤20 dB

Mild loss: 21–40 dB

Moderate loss: 41–70 dB

Severe loss: 71–90 dB

Profound loss: >90 dB

Case Studies

Case 1:

Presentation: A 5-year-old boy with speech delays, frequent earaches, and loud behavior. Audiometry revealed left-sided conductive hearing loss.

Diagnosis: Likely otitis media with effusion ("glue ear"), common in young children with peaks at 2 and 5 years.

Case 2:

Presentation: A 72-year-old woman with progressive hearing difficulties, mild tinnitus, and reliance on lip reading. Audiometry indicated bilateral sensorineural hearing loss.

Diagnosis: Presbycusis (age-related hearing loss), typically bilateral, symmetrical, and progressive in older adults.

Tympanometry

Definition

Tympanometry assesses middle ear compliance and pressure. Optimal sound transmission occurs when external and middle ear pressures are equal.

Procedure

1. A probe is inserted into the ear canal to produce sound, measure its reflection, and alter air pressure.

2. Pressure variations range from +200 mmH2O to -200 mmH2O, identifying the tympanic membrane's compliance.

3. Compliance peaks when no pressure difference exists across the eardrum.

Interpretation

Type A: Normal compliance with peak near 0 mmH2O. Variations indicate stiffness (e.g., tympanosclerosis) or flaccidity (e.g., ossicular disarticulation).

Type B: Flat trace, indicative of middle ear effusion or perforation (evidenced by elevated ear canal volume).

Type C: Negative pressure, suggesting Eustachian tube dysfunction.

Hearing Tests in Children

Otoacoustic Emissions (OAE)

Detects outer hair cell activity within the cochlea.

Used in neonatal screening programs to identify congenital hearing loss.

Presence of emissions indicates thresholds better than 40 dB.

Behavioral Techniques

1. 0–6 Months: Observe responses (e.g., movement, blinking) to auditory stimuli.

2. 6–18 Months:

Distraction Testing: Sounds are presented while the child is distracted by toys. A positive response involves the child turning toward the sound source.

Advanced Techniques

1. Visual Reinforcement Audiometry (9–36 Months):

Sounds are presented via speakers; correct responses are rewarded with visual stimuli.

2. Performance Testing (24–60 Months):

The child performs a task (e.g., placing a toy) upon hearing a sound.

3. Pure Tone Audiometry (≥5 Years):

Similar to adult testing, utilizing air and bone conduction assessments.

Comprehensive Overview of Otolaryngology Procedures

Grommet Insertion

Description

A grommet is a small ventilation tube designed to facilitate middle ear aeration. The procedure is typically conducted under local or general anesthesia.

Indications

Persistent otitis media with effusion lasting beyond three months.

Recurrent episodes of acute otitis media.

Retraction of the tympanic membrane due to compromised Eustachian tube function.

Technique

1. Position the patient supine on an operating table with the head turned laterally on a support ring.

2. Employ the largest aural speculum that fits comfortably to visualize the tympanic membrane through an operating microscope.

3. If necessary, remove any cerumen and assess the tympanic membrane for other conditions, such as cholesteatoma.

4. Perform a radial incision (myringotomy) in the safe antero-inferior quadrant of the tympanic membrane, suctioning any middle-ear fluid.

5. Insert the ventilation tube using crocodile forceps and position it with a Cawthorne hook or straight needle.

Postoperative Care

Performed as a day case; ensure ears remain dry for two weeks.

Audiological assessment is recommended 6–12 weeks post-procedure.

Grommets generally extrude spontaneously within 6–12 months, with tympanic membranes typically healing afterward.

Complications

Otorrhoea (ear discharge).

Tympanosclerosis (eardrum scarring).

Persistent tympanic membrane perforation (2–5%).

Middle Ear and Mastoid Surgery

Myringoplasty
A surgical intervention to repair tympanic membrane perforations, also termed Type I Tympanoplasty.

Tympanoplasty

Type II: Tympanic membrane reconstruction over malleus remnant and long incus process.

Type III: Reconstruction over the stapes head when malleus and incus are absent.

Type IV: Tympanic membrane reconstruction over the stapes footplate.

Type V: Involves stapes footplate fenestration due to fixation.

Type VI: Tympanic membrane reconstruction on the promontory.

Ossiculoplasty

Involves middle ear ossicle reconstruction.

Prostheses include TORPs (for absent stapes) and PORPs (for intact stapes head).

Materials: Hydroxyapatite, titanium, or bone cement for minor defects.

Mastoidectomy

Canal Wall Up: Combined Approach Tympanoplasty preserving the posterior ear canal wall.

Canal Wall Down: Modified radical mastoidectomy, removing the posterior ear canal wall.

Preoperative Care

Recent audiogram (within three months).

Ideally, ensure the ear is dry and infection-free.

Complications

Risks include infection, hearing loss, dizziness, tinnitus, taste disturbances (tympani injury), facial nerve damage, cerebrospinal fluid (CSF) leaks, and recurrence of disease.

Tonsillectomy

Indications

Chronic/recurrent tonsillitis.

Quinsy (peritonsillar abscess).

Obstructive sleep apnea.

Suspected malignancy.

Contraindications

Coagulopathy (manage with hematological input).

Acute infection, except for unresponsive quinsy.

Cleft palate due to potential velopalatal insufficiency.

Surgical Technique

1. Performed under general anesthesia with headlight illumination.

2. Patient positioned with neck extended using a shoulder roll.

3. A Boyle-Davis gag secures the mouth open.

4. Tonsils are excised by blunt or diathermy dissection, ensuring hemostasis.

5. Post-nasal suction clears potential obstructive clots before extubation.

Postoperative Care

Regular analgesia and early diet normalization.

Two-week recovery period advised.

Complications

Primary hemorrhage (within 24 hours).

Secondary hemorrhage (day 4–7).

Risk of infection, dental trauma, or temporary taste changes.

Adenoidectomy

Indications

Nasal obstruction with or without obstructive sleep apnea.

Recurrent otitis media.

Contraindications

Cleft palate or submucosal cleft.

Bleeding disorders.

Surgical Technique

Performed under general anesthesia, often alongside tonsillectomy or grommet insertion.

Adenoids are removed using suction diathermy or curettage under direct vision with an endoscope or mirror.

Complications

Risk of postoperative hemorrhage, dental injury, and transient speech changes.

Functional Endoscopic Sinus Surgery (FESS)

Indications

Chronic or acute sinusitis unresponsive to medical therapy.

Nasal polyposis, orbital complications, or sinus tumors.

Surgical Technique

1. Preoperative imaging (CT/MRI) aids in planning.

2. Performed with a zero-degree endoscope under general anesthesia.

3. Procedures include uncinectomy, ostium enlargement, and ethmoidectomy to restore sinus drainage.

Complications

Bleeding, nasolacrimal duct injury, numbness, orbital trauma, CSF leaks, anosmia.

Postoperative Care

Blood-tinged nasal discharge is common and self-limiting.

Saline douching and nasal steroid sprays are often prescribed.

Parotidectomy

Indications

Benign or malignant parotid gland tumors.

Surgical Technique

1. Performed under general anesthesia using facial nerve monitoring.

2. Incisions are made for adequate gland exposure, with care to identify and preserve the facial nerve.

Complications

Risks include bleeding, temporary or permanent facial weakness, hematoma, and sensory changes in the pinna.

Neck Dissection

Indications

Neck dissection is predominantly performed to manage metastatic carcinoma, often as part of treatment for head and neck cancers.

Types of Neck Dissection

1. Selective Neck Dissection (SND):

Involves the removal of specific lymph node groups (not all five levels).

Preserves all three non-lymphatic structures:

Sternocleidomastoid (SCM)

Accessory nerve (AN)

Internal jugular vein (IJV)

2. Modified Radical Neck Dissection (MRND):

Removes all lymph nodes from levels 1–5.

Retains one or more non-lymphatic structures, such as the SCM, AN, or IJV.

3. Radical Neck Dissection (RND):

Comprehensive removal of lymph nodes from levels 1–5.

Includes resection of the SCM, AN, and IJV.

4. Extended Radical Neck Dissection (ERND):

Builds on R&D by removing additional lymph node groups and/or other non-lymphatic structures, such as the external carotid artery or the posterior belly of the digastric muscle.

Consent and Complications

Patients should be informed about potential risks, including:

Bleeding or hematoma formation.

Infections at the surgical site.

Chyle leak due to lymphatic injury.

Nerve damage, including paralysis or sensory loss.

Facial lymphedema.

Recurrence of the primary disease.

Surgical Tracheostomy

Description

A tracheostomy is a surgically created airway via an incision in the neck and trachea. It can be performed either electively or emergently and may be temporary or permanent, depending on clinical need.

Indications

1. Airway obstruction:

Commonly addressed in emergencies (refer to ENT emergencies).

2. Ventilation support:

Reduces physiological dead space to aid in weaning patients from mechanical ventilation.

Facilitates tracheobronchial suctioning.

Surgical Technique

Performed under general anesthesia when possible, but local anesthesia may be used if endotracheal intubation is not feasible.

The patient is positioned supine with the neck extended using a shoulder roll and head ring.

Incision: A horizontal cut is made midway between the cricoid cartilage and the sternal notch.

Tissue Handling:

Strap muscles are divided and retracted.

The thyroid isthmus is either divided at the midline or partially transected.

Tracheal Opening:

A window or linear incision is made in tracheal rings 3 and 4.

The endotracheal tube is withdrawn, and the tracheostomy tube is inserted, ensuring its cuff is inflated.

Verification:

Confirm placement via CO_2 detection and bilateral lung air entry.

Secure the tube with tape and optional sutures.

Complications and Consent

Complications include:

Bleeding (intraoperative or postoperative).

Tube-related issues:

Dislodgment.

Blockage.

Formation of a false passage.

Infection.

Air leaks (subcutaneous emphysema, pneumothorax, pneumomediastinum).

Perioperative Care

1. Airway Maintenance:

Regular humidification and suctioning to prevent tube blockage.

Cleaning the inner tube.

2. Stoma Care:

Dressing changes and protecting surrounding skin.

3. Decannulation:

Considered once the tracheostomy is no longer essential.

Gradual downsizing and capping ensure patient tolerance.

Tracheostomy Tubes

1. Designs:

Most include inner and outer tubes. The inner tube is removable for cleaning, ensuring the airway remains open.

2. Fenestration:

Fenestrated tubes: Allow airflow for speech.

Non-fenestrated tubes: Speech may still occur if air leakage is sufficient.

3. Cuffed vs. Uncuffed Tubes:

Cuffed tubes: Essential for mechanical ventilation and aspiration prevention.

Uncuffed tubes: Used for non-ventilated patients with minimal aspiration risk.

Glossary

Adenoidectomy: Surgical removal of the adenoids, typically performed to address chronic infections or breathing difficulties.

Audiogram: A graph that represents an individual's hearing threshold at various frequencies and intensities.

Balloon Sinuplasty: A minimally invasive procedure to treat chronic sinusitis by widening sinus openings using a balloon catheter.

Cochlear Implant: An electronic medical device that provides a sense of sound to individuals with severe hearing loss.

Conductive Hearing Loss: Hearing impairment caused by a problem in the outer or middle ear that prevents sound from being conducted to the inner ear.

Endoscopic Sinus Surgery: A surgical technique using an endoscope to treat sinus problems, including chronic sinusitis and nasal polyps.

Epistaxis: Medical term for nosebleed, which may result from trauma, dryness, or underlying conditions.

Facial Nerve Paralysis: Loss of voluntary muscle movement in the face due to damage or dysfunction of the facial nerve.

Grommet Insertion: Placement of tiny tubes in the eardrum to relieve middle ear pressure or drain fluid.

Laryngoscopy: Examination of the larynx (voice box) using a laryngoscope for diagnostic or therapeutic purposes.

Mastoidectomy: Surgical removal of diseased mastoid air cells in the skull behind the ear to treat infections or complications from chronic otitis media.

Mixed Hearing Loss: Combination of conductive and sensorineural hearing loss, affecting both the middle and inner ear.

Neck Dissection: Surgical removal of lymph nodes and surrounding tissues in the neck, often performed for head and neck cancers.

Otosclerosis: Abnormal bone growth in the middle ear, leading to progressive conductive hearing loss.

Polypectomy: Surgical removal of nasal polyps, which are noncancerous growths in the nasal passage or sinuses.

Rhinoplasty: Surgical procedure to reshape or reconstruct the nose for functional or cosmetic purposes.

Sensorineural Hearing Loss: Hearing loss caused by damage to the inner ear or the auditory nerve.

Septoplasty: Surgical correction of a deviated nasal septum to improve airflow or relieve nasal obstruction.

Thyroidectomy: Surgical removal of all or part of the thyroid gland, often performed for thyroid disease or cancer.

Tonsillectomy: Surgical removal of the tonsils, usually to treat recurrent infections or obstructive sleep apnea.

Tracheostomy: A surgical procedure to create an opening in the trachea to bypass airway obstruction or facilitate long-term ventilation.

Vestibular Rehabilitation Therapy (VRT): A therapy designed to alleviate dizziness and balance disorders through customized exercises.

Zenker's Diverticulum: A pouch that forms at the back of the throat, leading to difficulty swallowing and regurgitation of food.

References

1. Bailey BJ, Johnson JT, Newlands SD. Head and Neck Surgery – Otolaryngology. 5th ed. Philadelphia: Lippincott Williams & Wilkins; 2014.

2. Bhattacharyya N. Clinical Essentials in Otolaryngology. 1st ed. Philadelphia: Elsevier; 2016.

3. Bluestone CD, Stool SE, Alper CM, et al. Pediatric Otolaryngology. 4th ed. Philadelphia: Saunders; 2003.

4. British Association of Otorhinolaryngologists – Head and Neck Surgeons (ENT UK). Standards and Protocols for ENT Practice. London: ENT UK; 2020.

5. Bull PD, Almeyda JS. Lecture Notes: Diseases of the Ear, Nose and Throat. 11th ed. Oxford: Wiley-Blackwell; 2018.

6. Cummings CW, Flint PW, Haughey BH, et al. Cummings Otolaryngology: Head and Neck Surgery. 7th ed. Philadelphia: Elsevier; 2020.

7. ENT UK. Guidelines for Tracheostomy Care in ENT Patients. London: ENT UK; 2021.

8. Gleeson M, Clarke RC. Scott-Brown's Diseases of the Ear, Nose, and Throat. 7th ed. London: Hodder Arnold; 2008.

9. Gormley WB, Grainger J, Wax MK. "Complications in Tracheostomy." Annals of Otology, Rhinology & Laryngology. 1999;108(2):140-145.

10. Johnson JT, Rosen CA. Bailey's Head and Neck Surgery: Otolaryngology Review. 6th ed.

Philadelphia: Lippincott Williams & Wilkins; 2014.

11. Kass JI, Anastasio AR. "Tracheostomy: A Surgical Perspective." Journal of Otolaryngology and Head-Neck Surgery. 2017;46:43.

12. KJ Lee, ed. Essential Otolaryngology: Head and Neck Surgery. 11th ed. New York: McGraw Hill; 2022.

13. Kountakis SE, ed. The Frontal Sinus. Berlin: Springer; 2005.

14. Lalwani AK. Current Diagnosis & Treatment Otolaryngology – Head and Neck Surgery. 4th ed. New York: McGraw Hill; 2020.

15. Maran AGD, Lund VJ. Clinical Rhinology. New York: Thieme; 2000.

16. Medscape. "Indications for Neck Dissection in Head and Neck Cancer." Medscape Reference. Updated 2022.

17. Myerson SG, Scott AD, Feyter PJ, et al. Imaging Techniques in Otolaryngology. Berlin: Springer; 2021.

18. National Institute for Health and Care Excellence (NICE). Hearing Loss in Adults: Assessment and Management. London: NICE; 2018.

19. Nicolai P, Castelnuovo P. Endoscopic Surgery of the Paranasal Sinuses and Anterior Skull Base. Berlin: Springer; 2015.

20. Oxford University Press. Oxford Handbook of ENT and Head and Neck Surgery. 2nd ed. Oxford: Oxford University Press; 2009.

21. Proops DW, Hawke M. Endoscopic Sinus Surgery: Anatomy, Three-Dimensional Reconstruction, and Surgical Technique. Edinburgh: Churchill Livingstone; 1993.

22. Robbins KT, Clayman G, Levine PA, et al. "Neck Dissection Classification Update by the American Head and Neck Society." Archives of Otolaryngology–Head & Neck Surgery. 2002;128(7):751-758.

23. Scott-Brown WG. Scott-Brown's Otorhinolaryngology, Head and Neck Surgery. 8th ed. London: CRC Press; 2018.

24. Tardy ME. Facial Aesthetic Surgery. 2nd ed. St. Louis: Mosby; 1997.

25. WHO. Hearing Care for All: A Guide for Policy Makers. Geneva: WHO; 2021.

26. World Health Organization (WHO). Prevention of Blindness and Deafness: Grades of Hearing Impairment. Geneva: WHO; 1991.

www.ingramcontent.com/pod-product-compliance
Lightning Source LLC
Chambersburg PA
CBHW071021240526
45469CB00006BD/2030